Cell Phones
and
The Dark
Deception

Cell Phones
and
The Dark
Deception

Carleigh Cooper

1st edition

ISBN: 978-0-578-00341-2

Premier Advantage Publishing
Copyright © 2009

Send information requests to:
contactus@premieradvantagepublishing.com
or
Premier Advantage Publishing
3819 Rivertown Pkwy., Ste 300-#210
Grandville, MI 49418
248.747.8234

Printed in the United States of America.

Dedication

This book is dedicated to my two beautiful daughters, both of whom have gone through the fire and have come out of it without smelling like smoke. I love you and am so proud of you, Jennifer and Holly. We have been through so much heartache together, but it's transformed us into the amazing women God wants us to be. To my late husband Steve, without whom this book would have never been written. I have always appreciated your loving kindness, your gentle spirit, and your continual support. I thank God that you're out of your misery and that you found your way home. And to my present husband, Keith, who has shown me how to live, love, and laugh again.

Also to all of our family and friends, who, for years, came alongside us to offer their unwavering love and support, even when they didn't understand what was wrong or know what to do. Special thanks to my mother, Susan; my father, Dave; my sister, Jane; Steve's parents, Don and Mary; my brother-in-law, Brian; my brother, Dean, and his wife, Janet; my step-sisters, Kathy and Theresa; and my dear friends - Kathy, Sylvia, Laura, Rebecca, Cindy, Joy, Mary, Laurie, and all the wonderful people at Harvest Fellowship who hugged us, loved us, and prayed for us during the times we needed it most.

Acknowledgment

The author gratefully acknowledges Janet Newton, President of The EMR Institute, for her assistance in editing this manuscript.

www.emrpolicy.org

Table of Contents

Preface

Hopeful. Yes, that's exactly what we were feeling. Hopeful. After years of searching and meeting with over thirty different doctors, neurologists and specialists, we finally met with one of the best toxicologists in the region. He conducted multiple tests on my late husband, Steve, and his exhaustive efforts were considered to be extremely thorough. The results were certain to reveal the disease or the source of the complications from which he suffered.

For over a decade no one had been able to diagnose or relieve Steve's myriad symptoms. Feelings of frustration and grief dominated, as we aggressively sought help and explored endless possibilities. It was vividly apparent that something was seriously wrong with him and he was only in his early forties. His health had been failing for years and it continued to decline; his ailments not only intensified, but new problems kept arising. The disconnected, but seemingly associated, symptoms made absolutely no sense to anyone.

As we anxiously waited for the toxicologist to enter the examination room in which we had been placed, I couldn't help but wonder about Steve's fate. Finally, the doctor came in and sat down across from us. He had a questionable smirk on his face as he reported that all of the test results had been received. Then he announced that he had good news. We were relieved, thinking, "Thank God he found something that wasn't too serious." That thought quickly faded when Dr. E proudly announced to Steve: "There's nothing wrong with you. No abnormalities were detected."

Dumbfounded, we sat there in disbelief. Steve's eyes grew big and his positive sense of hopefulness instantly shifted to anger. I can honestly say that in our 23 years of marriage, I had never seen so much rage bubbling up inside of him. He was usually mild-mannered. Without a doubt, it took every bit of restraint he had not to lunge at the doctor and grab his neck.

Instead, Steve lashed out verbally. "How can this be? How can all of these tests show absolutely nothing?" He wanted to know.

If you've ever been in a similar position, I don't have to tell you how devastating this kind of so-called "good news" is. It's heartbreaking to watch someone you love suffer agonizing pain day after day, month after month, and year after year. What's worse is when no doctor can help or determine what's wrong while your loved one is wasting away, you realize that there's not a damn thing you can do but pray. All you can see is a hopeless situation where there's no end in sight to your loved one's miserable existence.

Steve was a kind, gentle man and a loving father, who had become someone we no longer recognized. The unquenchable energy he once used to play with his girls had been completely drained from him. Always fatigued, he spent the majority of his time in bed. He suffered from chronic, excruciating, and debilitating migraine headaches. He was constantly hearing a wide variety of unusual sounds inside of his head, ranging from ringing and chirping to high-pitched screeching. The once peaceful, patient man was also overcome with feelings of anxiety, which were completely out of character. He'd become easily agitated, even angry at times for no apparent reason.

In addition, his previously sharp, intellectual mind had become foggy. He was extremely forgetful and often confused. Frequently, memories of close family, familiar people, places and events were no longer easily recollected. Likewise, understanding and following short stories, television programs, or in-depth conversations posed a challenge. Depression, accompanied by feelings of worthlessness and hopelessness, had also afflicted this once virile young man.

One year after seeing the aforementioned physician, it was recommended that we visit a well-known Neurotoxicologist in southern California. With Steve not working, it was a financial stretch, but we were promised it would be worth the trip. After all, Steve's problems were primarily neurological and he had been exposed to some toxic carcinogens at his previous job.

During the appointment we discussed the various chemicals Steve had been occupationally exposed to. There were only a couple that Steve recognized as being harmful, but few would have elicited the kind of complications he'd been experiencing. I asked the doctor if he was familiar with non-ionizing radiofrequency microwave (RF/MW) radiation and if he believed it was dangerous, because I needed to know if Steve's chronic close-range exposure to it could have been responsible for all or part of his disassociated gamut of symptoms. The Neurotoxicologist suggested that it was certainly a possibility, considering Steve's professional position.

As a technician, Steve spent 40+ hours a week building power microwave amplifiers for the base stations of cell towers. Every day for sixteen years, he was constantly being blasted in the face with RF/MW energy and, initially, the exposure was never considered as a probable cause of Steve's illness. After all, it was the same energy and technology that was incorporated into all wireless communication devices and that had never been shown to be dangerous...or had it?

Following the consultation, a series of tests were given. And even though we were sure that every possible exam had already been conducted, we were wrong. The outcome of both a TOVA test and a Brain Spect divulged the hidden secrets that had laid dormant deep within Steve's being. He finally received a diagnosis of Toxic Encephalopathy - brain damage due to toxic exposure. To our surprise, the areas of the brain that were damaged coincided precisely with each and every one of his abnormalities. It all made perfect sense.

"Now, what can we do to help him?" I eagerly asked. "What's next?"

The doctor fell silent and glanced down at the floor prior to answering. "There's really nothing that can be done," he said. "This disorder is progressive. It's not going to get any better." Then he added, "At this point, I recommend that you be watchful for the development of a brain tumor or brain cancer."

After three more years of anguish, on June 14, 2007, my dear, sweet Steve ended his life. He was only 48. It had become unquestionably evident to everyone around him that his health and mind were deteriorating to a point of no return. It had been a long, tough battle, during which he fought the good fight, but the illness overcame him. As an act of unfathomable desperation, he opted out. He had reached that absolutely horrific place, where there were no more options and there was nowhere else to turn; a place where all quality of life was lost and hope for anything better was gone.

My purpose for writing this book is multi-faceted. While I am not a scientist, nor do I claim to be an expert in this particular field, I have been led by life's experiences to explore this subject in great detail. If you've ever faced difficult circumstances, where help cannot be found, you know that you ultimately must rely on yourself to conduct a thorough investigation and find the answers you need. It doesn't take long to realize that no one cares about your situation as much as you do, so you have to be your own best advocate.

Believe me, if anyone had ever asked what topic I'd most like to study, given the time, I would have never said the effects of non-ionizing RF/MW radiation on the human body. I was not even familiar with the term. However, in the course of attempting to pinpoint Steve's source of aggravation, every other carcinogen that we knew he'd been exposed to had been ruled out. Through process of elimination, I began researching non-ionizing RF/MW radiation.

After months of reading through a multitude of credible studies, research papers, books, and other related literature, I was able to discover a great number of truths. Truths that, in my opinion, must be disclosed to the public. Our health is seriously being jeopardized, while the facts about cell phone dangers resulting from its RF/MW radiation exposure remain secret.

Living in blissful ignorance should no longer be an option for those who want to ascertain the definitive facts. *Cell phones have never been proven safe.* Like cigarettes, they were exempt from having to pass federally mandated FDA safety regulations. There are far more studies proving harm than safety when it comes to cell phones. I've invested 18 months into writing this book because there is no other document that addresses these dangers in such a clear, direct, comprehensible, and detailed format.

Furthermore, I strongly believe that all cell phone users have an undeniable right to know the risks they are taking every time they pick up their cell phones. I also believe that they have a right to learn how to protect themselves and their loved ones from harm.

I realize that Steve's exposure was greater than any you might experience. Nevertheless, research reveals that even the smallest injuries resulting from this type of exposure can accumulate and progress. In other words, prior to developing any permanent, recognizable damage from cell phone use, such as cancer, brain tumors, brain damage, or Alzheimer's disease, other adverse effects slowly and subtly creep in under the radar. It's so easy to fall into the trap of attributing frequent headaches, chronic fatigue, unprovoked anxiety, irritability, insomnia, concentration difficulties, and increased forgetfulness to stress. But is stress really the cause? Unfortunately, because of how the cell phone industry is governed in the United States, you are likely unaware that these are all common symptoms experienced by cell phone users.

As a dedicated spouse and father, Steve was involved in every aspect of our lives. The four of us, Steve, myself, and our two daughters, were very close and we spent the majority of our free time together. We enjoyed camping, hiking, canoeing, going to the lake, and visiting the park. Together, we attended every parent-teacher conference, talent show, 4-H affair, and sporting event our children took part in. Therefore, it's no wonder that these uninvited changes were not only difficult for Steve, but for all of us. They systematically invaded the man we loved and inadvertently destroyed our happy family. Our lives were forever transformed. Living that life of uncertainty, without help or hope, was the closest to Hell that I ever want to get.

Once one of Steve's treating physicians asked if I needed him to prescribe me some sort of medication to help me cope with everything that was happening and, after much contemplation, I chose to trust God instead of taking drugs. Although I already had a close relationship with the Lord, my focus of prayer had always been on Steve. I rarely prayed for myself, but that day I made a selfish and desperate plea on my own behalf. I cried out and asked God to take me out of the deep, dark pit I was drowning in and He answered my prayer the very next day. Whether you're a believer or not, impossible times call for a God who can do impossible things. Without Him as the foundation in our lives, I shudder to think where we'd be today.

In the eight months prior to Steve taking his life, God really did some miraculous things. Through His divine intervention my being was somehow altered. I was happy and at peace, even though our situation hadn't changed. He placed me in a wonderful women's Bible study class that, in reality, was a desperately needed support group. He not only brought me into a deeper relationship with Him, but He touched both of our girls with that same love and intimacy. Together, they chose to rededicate their lives to Christ. Additionally, Steve, who rarely attended church, asked to join us the Sunday before taking his life and during that service, he took that same step of faith. That in itself was a miracle.

Another reason for writing this book is that I refuse to accept that, for more than a decade, the four of us went through such tragic torment for nothing. Some good has to come out of it. And while a part of that "good" was growing stronger in our Christian faith, some of it should also be for the common good of others. Specifically, educating cell phone users on the real hidden dangers of cell phone use and RF/MW radiation exposure. Everything I've learned, you have a right to know. And as a Christian woman who is supposed to love her neighbor, how can I love you and not share this critical information with you?

Sadly, this information comes too late for many, who, like Steve, have been gravely deceived by the reality of this hazardous carcinogen. The truth is, cell phone use has never been proven safe. Some experts in this sphere of study even believe that the long-term illnesses endured by cigarette smokers will pale in comparison to those that will be experienced by cell phone users. If you're a cell phone user, get the facts. Don't wait until it's too late and don't allow the industry's propaganda or other misinformation to stand in the way of your continued good health and well-being.

You will soon discover why you're not hearing the whole truth. Educate yourself by reading this book. Knowledge is power. Without it you are defenseless against the chronic assault that you're receiving daily from your phone, other wireless connections, and the numerous cell towers in our environment. I guarantee that you will be enlightened and that you won't be disappointed.

With that being said, cell phones and their associated dangers remain a controversial issue. And, while most conclusions in this book are derived from credible insiders and scientific experts in the field, as a precautionary measure, it's imperative to state that the opinions and reasonable conclusions expressed by the author of this book may not reflect those of the publisher, wholesalers, distributors, and/or retailers.

CHAPTER 1

Where the Dark Deception Lies

According to the Cellular Telecommunications Industry Association (CTIA), at the end of 2006 there were over 224 million cell phone users in the United States.[1] Today that number has soared to more than 255 million.[2] What's even more phenomenal is the fact that, of the 6+ billion people on this planet, over one-third of them owns a cell phone and pays for service![3] There's no denying that the technology by which these phones operate is tremendous, or that the convenience and freedom they offer is beyond measure. Cell phones are wonderful and provide us with numerous benefits, but at what cost?

Over the past 24 years, cell phones have transformed dramatically. They began as bulky, "emergency only" bag units and they were unreliable. Furthermore, the geographical coverage was spotty. Yet, sales flourished. Today cell phones are no longer considered "emergency only" devices as initially intended and it's no longer uncommon to see 3 out of 5 people pressing a mobile phone to their ear, talking about anything and everything under the sun...whether or not the topic of discussion is important. Through industry design and promotion, they are now considered "must have" possessions; highly sought-after commodities of the modern age.

---

[1] *Insurance Information Institute*, http://www.iii.org (2008)
[2] CNN News, "Is There a Link Between Cell Phones and Cancer?", Larry King Live, 27 May 2008.
[3] Nystedt, Dan, "U.S. Marks New Cell Phone Record in 2005,". *IDG News Service*, 7 April 2006.

15

Today's phones are sleek; small enough to fit in your pocket, and capable of multiple functions. Aside from making a call, you can also access or accomplish any of the following: date book scheduling; download music; surf the Internet; send and receive text messages and email; take pictures and play games; record video footage; obtain navigational directions; and even watch television. Likely for these reasons alone, nearly every person over the age of 13 owns a cell phone. Those who don't are bound to feel the sting of social inadequacy.

However, since the popular device was first made available to consumers, cell phone users have questioned its safety. And though skepticism and controversy have continually challenged the wireless wonder, our growing attachment makes us quick to dismiss any negative information associated with its use, in favor of embracing that which is positive. Cells phones have become such an indispensable necessity that we yearn to believe they are safe.

Cell phone users are not the only ones who want to believe in cell phone safety. The industry, its manufacturers, and its service providers also want to convince you that their products are safe, primarily because they rely on close to $250 billion dollars in sales and service revenue each and every year. They've gone to great lengths to persuade you to accept the very notion of safety and continue to do so. They influence you in a variety of ways. They tell you what you want to hear and they keep the rest a secret.

This book is aimed at uncovering the deceptions and mysteries that have been taunting cell phone users for years. Your cell phone is probably important to you and you have grown dependent on it. You use it frequently and my guess is that you and your phone are literally attached at the hip. Let's face it, after reading this book, regardless what you learn, you're not going to give up your cell phone. Nor would I expect you to.

However, what will transpire is a deeper understanding as to (a) how cell phones operate; (b) how safety guidelines are established; (c) the role of the U.S. government in protecting its citizens; (d) industry regulatory and informational sources; (e) the results of worldwide cell phone related studies; and (f) the serious health hazards associated with wireless radiation exposure. You will also learn how to be smarter about using your cell phone; how you can easily protect yourself from unnecessary radiation exposure; and about how you are being deceived into believing that which is not true.

Deception *n.* the act of being deceived; to make a person or a group of people believe that which is not true; to intentionally mislead.

Deceptions are beliefs which are imposed with the deliberate intent to mislead or manipulate the truth. This type of dishonesty is often employed in order to change individual or group thought processes, actions, decisions, and behavior. Methods of persuasion can be verbal, nonverbal, or passively subtle, but whatever technique is implemented, the objective is always the same: to influence your belief system and cause it to fall in line with someone else's.

Unspoken persuasions and manipulations are often much stronger than those that are spoken or written. Subliminal messages like these can sneak into the subconscious, where they are often unknowingly and unwillingly accepted as truth. In other words, fiction is blindly embraced as fact when such a powerful belief system is imposed. You buy into it without question or realization of its acceptance and, while some deceptions pose no harm, others have dire consequences.

Deception Stems from Multiple Assumptions

Although the title of this book implies a single deception, there are actually many deceptions revolving around one core delusion - that cell phones are safe. The following misconceptions and deceptions seem to be most prevalent:

1. Cell phones are safe, with only a few exceptions.
2. Cell phone studies show no adverse health effects.
    (These studies, however, are typically conducted and funded by the cell phone industry.)
3. If cell phones are dangerous they would have never been mass marketed for consumer use and they wouldn't be as popular as they are today.
4. If cell phones are dangerous the government would surely protect its citizens from harm.
5. The only illnesses that have been remotely linked to cell phone use are brain cancer and brain tumors, and such incidents are rare.
6. Only chronic, abusive cell phone users are susceptible to health hazards; casual users are exempt.

17

7. If cell phone dangers truly existed the public would surely know.

As you will soon learn, what the majority of cell phone users believe to be true, isn't. Most of the information that makes up the foundation upon which these assumptions are based is secretly and intentionally hidden from consumers. It's time these truths were revealed and the facts disclosed. But the question is: Do you *really* want to know?

While discussing the topic of this book with family and friends, several cautioned that cell phone users wouldn't want to know the truth about cell phones and their related dangers. Conversely, others have sincerely thanked me for the information, saying that their eyes were opened and that they appreciated learning the truth, even though it wasn't what they wanted to hear.

Which category do you fall into? Do you really want to believe that cell phones are safe, even if they aren't? Do you want to allow yourself to be deceived or do you want to discover the truth? I firmly believe that knowledge is power and in order to be empowered, you have a right to know everything that I've learned over the past several years, even if you don't like it or agree with it. Discretion will protect you and understanding will guard you.

The Industry's Belief System

In his book, *Cellular Telephone Russian Roulette*, Dr. Robert Kane, a former Motorola engineer and a 30-year veteran of the telecommunications industry, proclaimed that, since the introduction of cell phones in 1984, the industry has developed and has instilled within us a "belief system," which has led us to accept the misconception that their phones are safe.[4] Cell phones would never be as popular as they are today if it wasn't for the industry's deep conviction, powerful persuasion, and ability to effectively impose their system of belief upon us.

Never in any multi-billion dollar cell phone media campaign has there ever been any mention of health risks, perceived or otherwise. The only observable risks derived from industry advertising are that you may not have enough minutes to talk as much as you want to or that your family might not have enough

---

[4] Robert Kane, *Cellular Telephone Russian Roulette* (New York, NY: Vantage Press, 2001), p. 191.

18

Book

phones to go around. The greatest risk of all is that you will be a social deviant if you don't own a cell phone. Sadly, this last hazard has effectively led millions of children, tweens (8-13), and teens into the fraudulent perception of threatened social acceptability. Ironically, cigarettes were marketed in this same manner. By smoking, one gained social acceptance and prestige; by choosing not to smoke, one would be put down, teased, or shunned.

To have an effective marketing strategy, the power of persuasion can best be implemented through frequency and repetition of impression. By repeatedly running the same ads or different ads with the same message over a long period of time, audiences are easily influenced. For a campaign to be successful, prospective consumers have to buy into and accept that which they are being "sold" and with enough financial support, this can easily be accomplished regardless of what the advertiser is selling - a product, service, concept or idea. Service providers like AT&T, Verizon, and Sprint usually concentrate on selling bigger and better calling plans, offering a greater number of monthly minutes. In doing so they're promoting the belief that it's okay to talk on your cell phone for that much time each month. What isn't said, but implied, is that you can do so without any risk of harm.

Likewise, by persuasively marketing family plans, the industry promotes the belief that it's just as safe for children to own and operate cell phones as it is for adults. And since these ads are intentionally designed to target both parents and children, parents are provoked into action, while their children are simultaneously prompted to request and eventually beg for the device that will elevate their popularity status. What the ads don't disclose is that multiple studies have shown that, because their brains are still developing, children and teens are much more susceptible than adults to the risks associated with microwave radiation, which is being deposited and absorbed more rapidly into their brains during cell phone use. To this day, the majority of Americans remain completely unaware that everything they are told about cell phones here in the U.S. is either industry promoted or industry approved. No opposing viewpoints are ever expressed because the government has given the telecommunications industry the authority and the undeserved right to govern itself.

Furthermore, no government funding is allocated for objective research. This effectively empowers the industry to suppress any potentially damaging information. While most

Americans rely on the media for accurate news and information, when it comes to cell phones, they are ignorant to the fact that the industry is the primary source feeding them their data. In essence, the media also plays a role in misleading the public.

In situations where an unbiased voice of truth is absent, consumers can become like sheep - easily led astray. You probably have no idea that researchers and experts in the field of electromagnetic radiation (EMR) and radiofrequency microwave (RF/MW) radiation, which is emitted from cell phones, perceive the cell phone industry as towing the same line the tobacco industry once towed. Only in this instance, they worry that the loss and destruction of life due to the former may exceed the latter. Even more important to consider is that it took over 100 years to gather enough scientific evidence for industry authorities to require the placement of warning labels on cigarette packages.[5] It is for this reason that I long to be a voice of truth in the issue of cell phone safety.

The Birth of Deception

When cell phones first became available for consumer use in 1984, they were widely embraced. Although there was little concern for safety at the time, the assumption was that they must be safe in order to be sold to the general public. It wasn't until 1993 that deception was deliberately birthed.

The cellular industry was hit with its first cancer lawsuit, which came as a complete shock to all cell phone users, and the negative publicity made the industry nervous and very defensive of their position on safety. The public's fear escalated, as did their health concerns, and cell phone stock began to plummet. But, instead of recognizing the incident as a possible red flag or as a warning of serious health issues to come, the industry panicked and focused solely on saving its reputation and protecting its assets.[6]

On ABC's 20/20 news broadcast, Paul Staiano, President of Motorola General Systems, responded to the accusations that cell phone use can cause cancer with a ridiculous exaggeration. He proclaimed that, "Forty years of research and more than 10,000

---

[5] George Carlo and Martin Schram, *Cell Phones: Invisible Hazards of the Wireless Age* (New York, NY: Carroll & Graf Publishers, 2001), p. 243.
[6] Ibid. pp. 6-9.

studies have proved that cellular phones are safe."[7] In an effort to provide evidence that this was in fact a true statement, the industry scrambled to compile documents that seemed to prove cell phone safety. Initially the studies presented appeared to be legitimate, but a closer look revealed that most, if not all of the data brought forth was derived from outside of the cellular frequency; not at all what cell phone users are exposed to. Therefore, the assertion that "more than 10,000 studies" proved safety was unmistakably invalid and clearly deceptive.

Because the media accepted the industry's statement as factual and publicized its claim without any evidence of validity, it wasn't long after the illegitimate news was released that public health concerns subsided and consumers experienced a newfound freedom to use their cell phones without fear of harm. After all, that's what every cell phone owner wanted to believe, that their phone was safe.

Following the 20/20 episode, Louis Slesin, editor of Microwave News and frequent industry safety critic, joined with others who accused the cell phone industry and its trade organization, the Cellular Telecommunications Industry Association (CTIA), of exaggerating research that supposedly supported claims of safety. An FDA official even went so far as to reprimand both the CTIA and the industry "for suggesting that enough scientific evidence exists to support the conclusion that cellular phones are safe".[8]

Consequently, by the time the truth was finally uncovered, the media exposure was remarkably less than that of the fraudulent safety statement previously made by the industry. Although the updated, more accurate information was undeniably controversial, it was definitely newsworthy, yet the message was never conveyed to the public. Why was it so easy for this information to be swept under the rug? Considering the history of publishing and advertising practices, the answer to that question is simple: Money, or rather, advertising revenue. If up to two-thirds of your income was derived from one key source, how likely would you be to destroy that relationship by exposing their faulty products and hindering the continued growth of their business? To do such a thing would be like slitting your own financial throat.

---

[7] Goldberg, Robert, "The Cellular Phone Controversy: Real or Contrived?," *EMF Health Report,* Vol. 1, No. 1, 1993.
[8] Keller, John, "Are They Safe?," *Wall Street Journal,* February 11, 1994.

Think about this for a minute. When you're watching television, reading the paper, surfing the Internet, or listening to the radio, you are constantly hammered with advertisements from five top industries: automotive; pharmaceutical; insurance; food service; and cellular service, not necessarily in that order. These advertising budgets equate to millions of dollars in media revenue annually, and, as we all know, money talks. The bigger the budget, the louder the voice. Recognize that each of these advertisers has substantial influence over the media venues with whom they choose to invest their billions.

This realization helps answer one of today's most prevalent questions which will be addressed further in the next chapter: "If cell phones are dangerous, why don't you know about it?"

A Reconciliation Attempt

After being caught in the lie that greatly deceived the American people, the wireless industry expressed regret over hastily claiming the untruth of cell phone safety as fact in a futile attempt to ensure self-preservation. As a follow-up effort to save its reputation and that of its products, the CTIA, the trade association representing cellular telephone service providers, hired the Wireless Technology Research Group (WTR) to conduct research on cell phone health and safety. Dr. George Carlo, director of WTR at the time, was to be paid up to $25 million dollars, over a three to five year period, to appease the public's uncertainty regarding any health concerns related to cell phone use. This was to be the world's largest research effort into wireless safety, during which Carlo was to prove once and for all that cell phones are not dangerous.

In the book, *Cell Phones: Invisible Hazards of the Wireless Age,* Carlo discloses that during his stint of employment with the WTR, he and his team conducted extensive research for the CTIA. Carlo believed the CTIA was confident that they had chosen someone to lead the research who could be won over if a situation should ever arise. But Carlo, a 39-year-old public health scientist, specializing in epidemiology from the George Washington University School of Medicine, was dedicated to acquiring the truth. He took his position of authority very seriously.

On December 3, 1998, Carlo reported to the CTIA that "it as unlikely that their mobile phones would cause health problems," but just 18 days later, that statement no longer held true.[9]

[9] George Carlo and Martin Schram, *Cell Phones: Invisible Hazards of the Wireless Age* (New York, NY: Carroll & Graf Publishers, 2001), pp. 14, 9, 149.

CHAPTER 2

The BIG Question

"If Cell Phones Are Dangerous, Why Don't You Know About It?"

There are some very valid reasons why you remain unaware of cell phone dangers associated with use. One is due to the fact that scientists and professionals in the medical and health industry don't see eye to eye on the issue of cell phone safety. Based on scientific knowledge, scientists understand the attributes of RF/MW energy and how it works. Likewise, health and medical experts base their opinions on knowledge relative to the medical field. Health experts focus on observing and evaluating how RF/MW energy interacts with and impacts the human body. In this way, they are better able to determine whether a danger or threat exists and what needs to be done in order to secure public safety. Both groups play an essential role, yet, because they approach the issue from differing viewpoints, they rarely share the same opinion.

Another reason it has been so difficult to arrive at a definitive answer to this question is that, even though experts review the same studies, they interpret the results differently. While many strongly believe that there is more than enough evidence to prove that adverse health effects exist from cell phone use, others are unwilling to admit any risk. The cause of this discrepancy is due to the fact that similar studies have not all arrived at consistent and identical outcomes. When assessing risk, some experts accept the results of short-term studies. Others however restrict their philosophies to only that which is derived from long-term, chronic exposure studies, of which there are few.

Additionally, some experts only take into account the effect that RF/MW radiation has on average, healthy people of median age, exempting those who are more vulnerable, such as those in poor health, children, pregnant women, and the elderly. This method of evaluation is inconceivable, not only because everyone has the right to be healthy and live quality lives, but because evaluation results cannot help but be skewed. Furthermore, now just about everyone on the planet has been exposed, so there is no longer a control group (those who have had no exposure) from whom the effects can be measured. Indeed, it would be extremely difficult, if not impossible, to conduct any type of long-term study of cell phone safety that would give an accurate account of how society is really being impacted.[10]

And last, but not least, the cellular industry is its own final authority and has ultimate control of whether the results of industry-funded studies, which make up the majority of research conducted in the U.S., are released or withheld from the public.

Who Are You Supposed to Believe?

Now that you understand why there is so much controversy among experts, let's move on to another pertinent question: "Who are you supposed to believe?" While considering this question, do you agree that inquiring information from a person or entity that has no third-party or monetary interest in the answer provided is the key to ascertaining the truth? Should you place your trust in those willing to share knowledge without hidden agendas or ulterior motives? Do you concur that it's always best to formulate opinions based on information provided by multiple independent sources, rather than on a few subjective ones? If you answered yes, permit me to assure you of two things.

First, that this book was written by such an individual; an informed, yet independent third party, who has been seeking the truth for her own benefit and who desires nothing more than to share what she has learned with you, because you have a right to know. My only motive is to help you discover the facts about cell phone radiation exposure and to assist you in obtaining real answers, which

---

[10] Sage, C., *The Bio Initiative Report,*
http://www.bioinitiative.org/report/docs/section_1.pdf (May 2008), p. 5.

will enable you to make wise decisions about your cell phone use, your health, and your future.

Second, that since most cell phone users are extremely skeptical and moderately sensitive about the subject of cell phone safety, this book relies on a compilation of information derived from multiple worldwide research efforts. The studies which will be shared with you have been conducted by an extensive array of extremely reliable and credible sources. These sources include, but are not limited to, various government agencies, highly respected and world-renowned scientists, biophysicists, epidemiologists, medical professionals, activists, scholarly individuals, and concerned organizations from all over the globe. Their discoveries will most certainly enlighten you, they may even shock you. Either way, their insight will provide you with enough evidence from which to draw your own conclusions concerning cell phone safety, or lack thereof.

Scientist Clas Tegenfeld, has studied the biological effects of electromagnetic fields (EMF) for years and he declares that, "already there are at least 15,000 scientific reports on the subject." While cell phone users are being told that not enough studies have been conducted and that there is no proof of harm, it is a known fact that cell phone radiation falls within the spectrum of electromagnetic radiation (EMR). Therefore, the effects are often similar. Tegenfeld feels that these studies offer more than enough scientific evidence to indicate risk. However, he is convinced that the findings are not being reported to consumers, because, "I'm afraid the truth is that we don't want to know". [11]

Dr. Neil Cherry, a leading physicist at Lincoln University in Canterbury, New Zealand, agrees, stating, "Strong claims by industry representatives and their consultants that there is no scientific evidence to justify the public's fears is scientifically, demonstrably wrong." In his numerous dose-response studies, Dr. Cherry proved that EMR exposure, such as the exposure from cell phones, is genotoxic, causes cancer, and has adverse health effects on the cardiac, reproductive and neurological systems. After extensive work in this field, he has concluded that the only safe level of RF/MW radiation, which is emitted from cell phones, cell phone towers, and other wireless connections, is *zero*! [12]

---

[11] Begich, Nick and Roderick, James, *Earthpulse Press, Inc.*, "Cell Phone Convenience or 21st Century Plague?," http://www.earthpulse.com/products/cellphoneplague.htm (July 2004).
[12] http://www.mapcruzin.com/radiofrequency/cherry/neil_cherry1.htm (2008).

Likewise, Dr. Robert Kane, who spent 30 years working in the telecommunications industry and has a Ph.D. in Electrical Engineering, calls attention to revelations that have been established over a 45-year span. Between 1950-1995, there has been confirmed, solid evidence proving three truths about cell phones and those who promote their use. The first is that cell phones expose operators to dangerous and highly destructive levels of radiofrequency energy, which is bodily absorbed. Second, cell phone manufacturers, service providers, governments, and scientists have long been aware of the hazards. And finally, that the previously mentioned entities have not warned cell phone owners of the hidden dangers.[13]

These yet to be disclosed statements may be difficult to accept, but if all of these statements are true, the original question: "If cell phones are dangerous, why don't you know about it?" remains.

The Government's Role

It may surprise you to learn that, prior to cell phones being mass marketed to the general public, there was never any government mandated pre-market testing to certify that they were safe to use. Pre-market safety testing by the FDA (Food & Drug Administration) is mandatory for every consumer product that will be purchased and utilized in the U.S. Food, drugs, beauty products, children's toys and any other item distributed to the general public must be safety tested and approved prior to its release. But for some obscure and questionable reason, cell phones were neither tested nor scrutinized to ensure safety prior to their release. Without any safety assurances whatsoever, the U.S. government gave the cellular industry the "green light" to sell their radiation-emitting devices to unsuspecting buyers; a trusting population that assumes adequate government protection.

In the book, *Cell Phones: Invisible Hazards of the Wireless Age*, Dr. George Carlo, chief scientist of the world's largest research effort into wireless safety, expressed frustration with the government's decision. He was appalled to realize that in the year 2000, with over 100 million cell phone owners in the U.S., the government had still done nothing to protect its citizens from the hazardous risks that remain secret from the public. Now, with over

---

[13] Robert Kane, *Cellular Telephone Russian Roulette* (New York, NY: Vantage Press, 2001), p. 40.

255 million cell phone users in the U.S., your safety continues to be jeopardized, as cell phones remain an untested and unregulated consumer product.[14]

The Federal Communications Commission (FCC) is a licensing and engineering agency that oversees the development and use of communications technology. It does not test, fund, or conduct research on cell phones, cell towers, or the microwave radiation emitted from them. The FCC relies on the cellular industry to govern and monitor itself for compliance. Moreover, the FCC admits that it does not have the knowledge or expertise to determine radiation exposure guidelines for safety. Therefore, they have entrusted three independent engineering organizations - the Institute of Electrical and Electronic Engineers (IEEE), the American National Standards Institute (ANSI), and the International Commission on Non-ionizing Radiation Protection (ICNIRP) – to determine safe exposure levels for the nation.[15]

Quoting an FCC official in 1994, the Bloomberg News Service confirmed the previous statement: "The FCC is not in the business of doing basic biological research to ascertain how cell phones might affect the brain." Dr. Robert Cleveland, cellular biologist and former director of the FCC's office of engineering and technology, also established the agency's disregard in the area of research and testing by saying, "We (the FCC) don't have the authority to do that sort of thing. The FDA is more in line to do that kind of thing."

However, later that same year, the FDA did mandate the FCC to require all cell phone manufacturers to certify that their products meet safety standards. But again, no government agency or authoritative entity oversees or ensures that cell phones actually do adhere to those definitive certification requirements. The government simply trusts manufacturers to fulfill that obligation. By the same token, the FDA also admits that it does not review or test any radiation-emitting devices, such as wireless phones, for safety. Not only does the FDA not test radiating-emitting devices, but they admit

[14] George Carlo and Martin Schram, *Cell Phones: Invisible Hazards of the Wireless Age* (New York, NY: Carroll & Graf Publishers, 2001), p. 77.
[15] Brown, Gary, *Wireless Devices, Standards, and Microwave Radiation in the Education Environment,* http://www.emfacts.com/wlans.html, (October 2000).

29

to having no regulatory authority to require manufacturers to conduct long-term product studies in order to ensure long-term safety.[16]

An Opportunity to Alert the Nation

In the summer of 2000, Dr. David Feigal, the FDA's Chief of the Center for Devices and Radiological Health, appeared on the CNN news program, *Larry King Live*. This branch of the FDA is a consumer watchdog that's responsible for alerting the public of suspected threats whenever they arise. According to Dr. George Carlo, just seven days earlier Feigal's agency hosted a conference, during which Motorola's scientist, Dr. Joseph Roti Roti revealed his most recent findings. Roti Roti informed the FDA and others at the conference that cell phone radiation caused genetic damage to human blood cells. But instead of sharing this deeply concerning information with King's millions of viewers, Feigal chose to side with the industry in misleading the public into believing that cell phones pose no health risk.[17]

In a letter dated January 16, 2001, Feigal commented: "We don't have the money to protect consumers from wireless technology".[18] With that being said by an insider, it clearly establishes the fact that neither the FCC nor the FDA is sufficiently protecting the health and well-being of American citizens. Coincidentally, this observation was reiterated later the same year inside the walls of a Louisiana Federal District Court, when it was concurred that the public could not depend on either FCC or the FDA for protection against RF/MW radiation exposure.[19]

Who Governs the Giants?

With no government safety assurances in place or funding available for objective, third-party research, you are in an extremely vulnerable position. By default, you are left to rely on a biased, subjective industry that feeds on your ignorance for their economic

[16] George Carlo and Martin Schram, *Cell Phones: Invisible Hazards of the Wireless Age* (New York, NY: Carroll & Graf Publishers, 2001), pp.78-80.
[17] Ibid. pp. 229-230.
[18] Silva, Jeffery, "FDA Ill-Equipped for Health Issue," *RCR News*, February 19, 2001.
[19] Brown, Gary, *Wireless Devices, Standards, and Microwave Radiation in the Education Environment*, http://www.emfacts.com/wlans.html, (October 2000).

livelihood, to ensure your safety. To your detriment, there has never been any organized opposition to refute these political decisions. This wrongful exchange of authority has empowered the cellular industry to deceive you into believing whatever it is that they choose to tell you about their products and service. They, after all, are their own final authority.

Why Are There So Many Contradicting Reports?

The answer to this question can be narrowed down to three key elements: industry control, industry preservation, and global truths. Inconsistencies develop when industry control and preservation collide with global truths. As you can well imagine, the cellular industry does not want conflict or questions from the public or the media regarding the safety of cell phones.

Whenever industry funding *is* made available and industry researchers present unfavorable results, funding is often cut and all supporting documentation is conveniently destroyed. This is why there is such a small number of negative reports emerging from the U.S. Few researchers are willing to stand up to the cell phone industry and jeopardize their livelihood. They are fully aware that they could be fired or discredited for not providing their employer with the results they paid for.

To further insure industry control and preservation, other protective measures are taken when scientific evidence proves harm or initiates controversy. Any threatening news that cannot be contained prompts CTIA representatives to "spin the truth" to their advantage. This has long been an effective way to hold public relations to specific standards. Anything derogatory is rejected and depicted as fictitious, rather than fact, when thought to have damaging effects.

Hollywood celebrities, politicians, and large corporations, including both the tobacco and cell phone industries, all hire public relations professionals to employ these influential, image preserving techniques when necessary. According to insider Dr. Kane, CTIA seminars even go so far as to, "teach cellular industry people how to wage the public relations battle for the minds of the public".[20] Doing this enables them to consistently maintain and project their belief system of safety to consumers. Reports that contradict the

---

[20] Robert Kane, *Cellular Telephone Russian Roulette* (New York, NY: Vantage Press, 2001), p. 234.

information received from the industry generally come to U.S. consumers from other countries.

Industry Concealment

As previously mentioned, the WTR, operating under the direction of Dr. George Carlo, was established by the industry (CTIA) in 1993 to conduct independent research to prove safety. However, within a relatively short period of time during which numerous studies were conducted, there arose serious reason for concern. Because the findings were so disturbing, studies were repeated, but even varied techniques produced similar results. To insure validity, three groups of world-renowned scientists had the studies peer-reviewed by independent experts. After much scrutinizing, the WTR confirmed that cell phone radiation causes genetic changes in human blood cells.

It has long been widely recognized and accepted that all tumors and cancers are the result of genetic damage. This same kind of damage resulted when human blood cells were exposed to wireless signals from all types of phones: analog, digital, and PCS. Following exposure, there was also evidence of multiple cells with micronuclei in the human blood. The development of micronuclei (many nuclei, rather than one nucleolus) in the blood is one of the best indicators of cancer risk, as well as other health hazards. It identifies cells which are no longer able to repair their broken DNA.

At current exposure levels, cell phone users remain particularly vulnerable to these hazardous developments.

Those at the WTR were alarmed by the findings and as you can imagine, the news did not sit well with industry leaders. Following his research, Carlo immediately addressed the CTIA about devising a new, more realistic safety exposure standard for radiation emissions from cell phones. He informed Jo-Anne Basile, vice president of the CTIA, of the crisis, telling her that it was shameful and that the industry was failing to meet its public health responsibility by willfully exposing cell phone users to harmful emission levels. Reportedly, her response to him was, "How dare you talk to us like that after all the money you've been paid?"[21]

---

[21] George Carlo and Martin Schram, *Cell Phones: Invisible Hazards of the Wireless Age* (New York, NY: Carroll & Graf Publishers, 2001), pp. 6, 149-154.

After this, the WTR's research funding was cut. Researchers hired by the industry encounter complex situations when results challenge or negate the belief system of safety. Carlo was not alone in his efforts to definitively speak out about the adverse health effects that his research team discovered. Other experts in the field, including Dr. Ross Adey, Dr. Jerry Phillips, and Dr. Henry Lai, have also refused to be bought by the industry.

While working for Motorola, Dr. Ross Adey, one of the world's most respected and widely published RF senior researcher from the University of California, Riverside, had his funding immediately terminated when he revealed that mobile phone emissions significantly increased the number of brain tumors in animals. His research also reiterated the findings of many other studies proving that these same emissions cause DNA damage. Dr. Jerry Phillips, Adey's associate at the time, said that their working relationship with Motorola was pleasant prior to disclosing their conclusions. Afterward, tensions were stretched. Phillips asserted that, "Motorola was adamant that Adey never mention DNA damage and RF radiation in the same breath." [22]

The irresponsible decision not to disclose the truth about the impact their phones have on consumers was so disheartening that Adey chose to expose the truth of what happens inside the industry and how research procedures are inappropriately managed. He confessed that, "Motorola has been manipulative of research that we and others have reported to them. Essentially, they cut us off, because we were too inquisitive." Motorola was unwilling to hear, let alone accept anything derogatory regarding their phones. [23]

Phillips shared Adey's concern and likewise revealed Motorola's displeasure with their study's concluding report. He even divulged the fact that the manufacturer was looking for ways in which they could "spin" the findings to project them in a more positive light. These were not the kind of outcomes they had paid for or were looking to obtain. Therefore, Motorola was unwilling to accept what these leading experts had determined as fact. They even urged Phillips not to publish the results, but recognizing the incredible magnitude of their research, Phillips disregarded

---

[22] Fleming, "Cover-Up Claims Over Mobile Phone Danger," *Express Newspapers*, May 24, 1999.

[23] Begich, Nick and Roderick, James, *Earthpulse Press, Inc.*, "Cell Phone Convenience or 21st Century Plague?," http://www.earthpulse.com/products/cellphoneplague.htm (July 2004).

Motorola's request and made known what was meant to remain secret.[24]

Then, there are Dr. Henry Lai's research findings to take into account. After 20 years of research for the industry, Lai, a top bioelectromagnetics researcher at the University of Washington, Seattle, and his colleague, N.P. Singh, observed DNA strand breaks in rats after they had been exposed to electromagnetic fields similar to those cell phone users are exposed to. Lai was quoted in the London Times as saying: "They are asking me to change my whole interpretation of the findings in a way that would make them more favorable to the mobile phone industry. This is what happened in the tobacco industry. They had data in their hands, but when it was not favorable, they did not want disclose it." [25] Instead they hid the truth, just as the wireless industry is doing.

Both doctors, Adey and Lai, are not unrecognized in the fields of microwaves and radiation. In fact, they are two of the world's leading scientific experts. They have both been involved in multiple research projects, including military ones, and their expertise concerning the health effects of EMF (electromagnetic fields) has been employed to increase the military's understanding of potential weapon applications. Thanks to their integrity and autonomy, we can trust their repetitive and firmly established findings.[26] And, even with their solid backgrounds in scientific research, both experts share similar working experiences when it comes to the inside operations of the cell phone industry.

Adey, Phillips, Lai, and others see a strong parallel between what is happening now and the decades of denial by the tobacco industry. Just as the tobacco industry withheld harmful information from the public, the cell phone industry is following suit. In fact, in a December 1994 internal Motorola memo, Motorola Inc. devised a plan to collaborate with the Cellular Telecommunications Industry Association (CTIA) and Wireless Technology Research L.L.C.

---

[24] Kelley, Libby, CWTI (Council on Wireless Technology Impacts), and EON International, DVD *"Public Exposure: DNA, Democracy and the Wireless Revolution",* 2000.
[25] Health Effects of Microwave Radiation (Western View),
http://www.Goodhealthinfo.net/radiation/health_efx_western.htm
[26] Begich, Nick and Roderick, James, *Earthpulse Press, Inc.,* "Earth Rising- The Revolution: Toward a Thousand Years of Peace," http://www.earthpulse.com (January 2000).

(WTR) to downplay any potentially damaging scientific findings on possible health risks from portable telephones.[27]

These are prime examples from three industry-hired research experts and their experiences which are indicative of what happens to industry-funded studies that evoke unfavorable results. "It's all about science, politics, and money, and not necessarily in that order," says Dr. Louis Slesin, editor of Microwave News. "Henry Lai and N.P. Singh had the courage to buck the system, and they have paid dearly for that." Lai and others say that funding from the industry can come with restrictions so oppressive they hamper scientific inquiry.[28]

When it comes to manipulating research, Joseph Hotchkiss of Cornell University has commented on the ease of changing undesirable or threatening industry conclusions. "A host of techniques exist for manipulating research protocols to produce studies whose conclusions fit their sponsor's predetermined interests. These techniques include adjusting the time of a study (so that toxic effects do not have time to emerge), subtle manipulations of target and control groups or dosage levels, and subjective interpretations of complex data. Often such methods stop short of outright fraud, but lead to predictable results. Usually, associations that sponsor research have a fairly good idea what the outcome will be, or they won't fund it."[29]

Dr. Jerry Phillips sums up the truth of industry-funded research in these words, "To buy a study is to be sure that your billions of dollars are safe".[30]

---

[27] Begich, Nick and Roderick, James, *Earthpulse Press, Inc.,* "Cell Phone Convenience or 21st Century Plague?,"
http://www.earthpulse.com/products/cellphoneplague.htm (July 2004).
[28] Harrill, Rob, "Wake-up Call," *Columns,* The University of Washington Alumni Magazine, March 2005.
[29] Maisch, Don, "Mobile Phone Use: It's Time to Take Precautions," *Journal of the Australasian College of Nutritional and Environmental Medicine,* Vol. 20, No. 1, April 2001.
[30] Kelley, Libby, CWTI (Council on Wireless Technology Impacts), and EON International, DVD *"Public Exposure: DNA, Democracy and the Wireless Revolution",* 2000.

Following the evidence that cell phone radiation has been repeatedly shown to cause DNA damage, "Dr. George Carlo, in his capacity as director of WTR, wrote a letter to the CEO of AT&T which has serious legal implications for mobile phone manufacturers who have claimed that there is no evidence for adverse health effects from mobile phone use. With the letter widely circulated in the industry, making *that* claim now could possibly expose them to litigation in much the same way as what happened to the tobacco industry, where it was shown that industry assurances of no evidence of hazards from smoking was a complete fabrication."[31]

Isn't it ironic that expert researchers who have been employed by the cellular industry for a number of years are comparing this cover up of truth to that of the tobacco industry? Consider the number of years and the hundreds of thousands of lives that were destroyed or lost, before the tobacco industry finally came clean. Even today there are commercials reporting that 1,200 people a day continue to die from smoking-related diseases.[32]

As with other carcinogenic exposures such as asbestos, lead paint, pesticides, and the like, it can take 25-30+ years of research before there is sufficient "proof" of harm. Consider the fact that 100 years passed, before a warning was mandated for placement on cigarette packs.

Due to this extended period of time, the link between cell phones and the associated dangers resulting from microwave radiation exposure may not be made known to the public until it's too late. What makes this sequence of events significantly worse than that of the tobacco industry is that it's not only cell phone users who are at risk, but everyone's health is being jeopardized. Hundreds of thousands of cell phone antennas and relay towers are spread across this great nation and every second of every hour of every day, they are constantly transmitting signals. This means that our bodies are chronically being assaulted by invisible beams of RF/MW radiation, and this unnatural, radiant energy is being absorbed into our bodies, causing serious health problems.

---

[31] Maisch, Don, "A Letter Bomb for the Mobile Phone Industry?," *EMFacts Consultancy*, October 19, 1999.
[32] *Truth ads*; http://www.thetruth.com (2008).

CHAPTER 3

A Desperate Search for Answers

Our catastrophic, life-changing story began in November 1995. At the age of 36, my late husband Steve was finally convinced to visit a doctor. He had been dealing with chronic headaches for months and had been downing aspirin as if they were candy. As with most people, for lack of a better explanation, Steve quickly attributed his excruciating headaches to work and stress. Blurred vision, nausea, insomnia, fatigue, ringing in the ears, anxiety, memory loss and confusion soon accompanied his headaches. Mood swings, irritability, and depression just as eagerly joined in. When the pain became too intense in March of 1999, my spouse of 15 years was no longer able to work; he spent most of his time in bed.

By 2001, Steve had seen more than 30 different doctors, neurologists, and specialists, all who had tried to help, but failed. Numerous tests had been initiated and various drugs prescribed; yet no relief was found. Steve remained sick, undiagnosed, and unsure of the path his life was taking. His symptoms were unrelated and made no sense whatsoever to any of the experts we met with. Within a relatively short period of time, each would inevitably reach a point of frustration where they were no longer able to offer any suggestions, prescriptions, direction, referrals, or hope.

The drive home after these particular doctor visits was always silent. Tensions were high and our level of aggravation mounted. It became increasingly apparent that if we were going to get any answers *we* would have to find them ourselves.

It was after yet another one of these disappointing visits that I could no longer remain silent on the ride home. We had been through so much, but I was not willing to give up without a fight.

Steve on the other hand, faced the daily struggle of just trying to cope and, after 6 long years he had little fight left in him. He was understandably tired and ready to surrender. I however, was unwilling to allow him to accept defeat. I looked intently at my partner in pain and began shooting off rapid-fire questions at him.

One right after another I fired flaming arrows of interrogation his way. The inquiries were all about the job he had held for the past 16 years. I persistently demanded to know everything: what he had done and how he done it; what kind of chemicals, products, or other dangerous toxins he'd been exposed to; and anything else he could remember. I was sure that if we were able to target some potential causes of his illness, we could make some sort of connection. In doing that, we'd be able to get Steve some desperately needed help. I knew very little about his job; he was restricted from talking about it and I had only been inside his workplace once, on Visitor's Day. Knowing that he had been issued top security clearance for his important position didn't hinder me from proceeding in the least bit. After all, I wasn't searching for top security information. I just wanted to know what was destroying my husband.

I was determined to learn why he continued to suffer from chronic and debilitating headaches, years after leaving work. I wanted to know why no medical professional could assist and why no prescription drug offered any relief. I wanted to ascertain why he behaved so erratically at times without being provoked. It was important for me to discover why, at age 42, he was so forgetful, why he was so frequently confused and disoriented, and why he was incessantly fatigued and depressed.

The Search Begins

Making sense of the answers Steve provided posed a definite challenge, because every word that came out of his mouth sounded foreign to me. He was spewing out terms like radiofrequency and non-ionizing microwave radiation, as if their meanings were common knowledge. With a deep sense of urgency I began an intense search on the Internet, using the phrase "radiofrequency non-ionizing microwave radiation", and in the advanced search field I typed in the exact phrase, "adverse health effects." It was baffling not only to see the number of results, but also that almost every one of them referred to cell phones and their related dangers.

Confused and irritated because that wasn't the type of information I was seeking, the search was deleted and repeated. Despite a number of attempts using various phrases, the results remained the same. I was certain that something was wrong with the search engines I was using, because "cell phone dangers" was not the category I was looking for. After all, I had owned a cell phone since 1989 and, to my knowledge, there had never been any proof of danger. I, like everyone else, believed they were safe.

The only potential danger I was aware of was the remote possibility that chronic cell phone use could cause brain tumors or brain cancer, but casual users were unaffected. Furthermore, evidence of this had never been substantiated.

But since multiple searches kept providing similar results, I chose to visit and read through some of the web sites, though the possibility of finding what I was looking for seemed unlikely. I figured it couldn't hurt.

I was soon surprised to discover that the information I had stumbled upon made a whole lot of sense. Among other things, I learned that cell phones utilize radiofrequency non-ionizing microwave radiation to transmit and receive wireless signals, clearly indicating a relationship between Steve's employment and cell phones. Specifically, the microwave power amplifiers that he had built and tested for years were being used in the base stations of cell towers all over the world. They were also being utilized to facilitate satellite communications, radar operations, and military weapon applications. All of these and other wireless communication signals operate using the same microwave radiation to perform messaging functions. As the pieces of the puzzle started coming together, I was eager to learn more.

Radiofrequency Microwave (RF/MW) Radiation

All wireless communication signals are transmitted and received using radiofrequencies of various power levels and wave lengths. What began with the wireless broadcasting of radio and television has exploded into an array of new technologies that have changed the world. Cell phones, cordless phones, pagers, radar, wireless Internet, and satellite communications all operate using different radiofrequencies at the microwave level.

Typically when one hears the term "microwave", they reference that which is most familiar: microwave ovens. That being recognized, there are three principle differences between the microwaves used for wireless signaling and those used in microwave ovens: frequency, power, and heat. Although the microwave range is quite vast, these elements determine the characteristics of microwaves. For example, the series of frequencies at which cell phones operate span from 750 to 950 MHz (mega hertz). Microwave ovens however, operate at a much higher frequency of 2450 MHz. While microwave ovens use high frequency and high power, cell phones operate using high frequency and low power.

Heat is the third differentiating factor between the microwave radiation used to operate cell phones and that which is used in microwave ovens. While both of these devices elicit the same type of heat, that heat does not generate the same response. The RF/MW radiation used in microwave ovens produces an intense, detectable heat that cooks food. In contrast, the heat which is generated from cell phone microwave radiation is rarely perceived externally. Although it is powerful enough to cook, it does so from the inside out and rarely heats the surface. The heating effect from these microwaves takes place deep within the human tissue and goes undetected. This absence of heat presents us with another cell phone deception, as you will soon discover.

Unfortunately, to our detriment the latter heating concept is much more difficult to grasp. This is due to the fact that the deep tissue heating which transpires inside of the brain of a cell phone user from its microwaves is rarely felt on the skin's surface, where the phone is held. It's not until the microwave energy is deposited, absorbed, and converted into heat well below the epidermal layer that dangerous temperature increases take place and damage occurs. Temperature increases associated with absorption have been shown to occur within the first 60-90 seconds of exposure. In other words, after being on your cell phone for as little as 60 seconds, damage can start to take place. Even though you seldom feel warmth while talking on your phone, at the point where heat is detected, brain damage is already occurring. What's worse is that the brain has no pain receptors to warn you of the severity of such an injurious assault.

Without any heating sensation whatsoever, you may have trouble accepting the fact that cell phone microwaves have been proven to cook brain tissue much more quickly and efficiently than a microwave oven. Consider this: if it only takes 60-90 seconds of microwave oven radiation to boil one cup of water, and if cell phone microwaves cook more quickly and efficiently, and your brain is 90% water, imagine what's happening to your brain after a 60-90 second phone call. [33]

Ionizing vs. Non-Ionizing Radiation

In order to fully comprehend the dangers posed by cell phones, cell towers, and other wireless devices, and to understand the basis upon which U.S. safety standards are established, it's essential that you be able to distinguish between the two types of microwave radiation - ionizing and non-ionizing. Ionizing radiation is made up of very short electromagnetic waves of very high frequency and is located at the upper end of the electromagnetic spectrum. This type of radiation is referred to as "ionizing" because its energy travels at such extremely high speeds that tightly bound electrons detach from their pre-existing union with atoms. This breaking of chemical bonds creates ions, or electrically charged atoms, which emit radiation.

Ionizing radiation exists naturally in the form of solar energy, cosmic rays, and radioactive elements found in the earth. This power source includes gamma rays; it has also been integrated into man-made applications such as x-ray technology and that which is used to generate electric and nuclear power. This form of radiation is universally recognized as being harmful and biologically interactive. Exposure penetrates the human body causing injury to living tissue, skin burns, and a variety of other adverse reactions including genetic damage and cancer.

Conversely, non-ionizing radiation is made up of longer electromagnetic waves operating at lower frequencies; these signals are weaker, therefore they reside closer to the bottom of the electromagnetic spectrum. Examples of non-ionizing radiation in sequence of power begin with low energy emissions from power lines, they include RF radio and television broadcast signals, and the high end is comprised of microwave ovens and microwave energy which is used to operate all forms of wireless communication. Since microwaves reside so close to ionizing radiation, their power has the greatest intensity of all non-ionizing radiation forms.

Like ionizing radiation, microwaves are made up of very short (micro) and powerful electromagnetic waves of high frequency, but they are not powerful enough to become ionized. Non-ionizing

---

[33] Robert Kane, *Cellular Telephone Russian Roulette* (New York, NY: Vantage Press, 2001), pp. 6, 12-14.

radiation in this upper range of the electromagnetic spectrum is generally referred to as radiofrequency microwave (RF/MW) radiation, cellular radiation, and electromagnetic radiation (EMR).

As previously mentioned, heat, power, and frequency are the attributes that determine the conduct of microwaves; their differences in these three areas have also been established. Therefore, it seems extremely unreasonable that microwave ovens are paired with cell phones on the electromagnetic spectrum when they are obviously poles apart.

In the developmental stage, cell phones were thought to be harmless because the only perceived dangers from microwaves were those associated with heating and cooking. Since pressing a cell phone against one's head doesn't cause any immediate burning sensation, discomfort or pain, the industry and those who determine safety standards presumed them to be safe. Scientists were also convinced that, while cell phones operate using low power and microwave ovens operate using high power, chances of any adverse health effects from cell phone use were slim to none. They even developed a synchronized understanding that unless radiation was able to produce internal temperature increases enough to elicit whole body heating there was absolutely nothing to worry about.

When it comes to cell phone safety, U.S. guidelines, which have been put into place for our protection from non-ionizing RF/MW radiation, continue to be based on these same preconceived notions. Standard setters continue to base safety on the outdated premise that, if radiant energy doesn't heat the entire body and raise internal body temperature, it can't be harmful. This principle has remained in effect even though science has repeatedly proven that non-ionizing microwave radiation causes deep bodily tissue damage from heating without raising internal body temperature. When it comes to safety, maintaining this archaic theory is irresponsible.

To enhance your understanding of the ridiculous foundation upon which our so-called safety standards are based, consider the following examples. If you hold your finger over a flame, it will begin to get hot and is likely to burn (adverse health effect). If you are out in the sun too long without protection, you are also likely to burn (adverse health effect). These adverse health effects (external burns) are likely to result without increasing your overall internal body temperature and, according to the premise upon which safety exposure standards are founded, if heating doesn't produce a total body temperature increase of at least 1° Celsius (equivalent to an internal increase of 1.9° Fahrenheit), exposure can't be harmful. And, as with these examples of direct exposure, similar results occur from cell phone RF/MW radiation when holding the device up against the head. The undetected heat from the exposure is not evenly absorbed or distributed throughout the human body; therefore it is impossible to cause a total body temperature increase, yet exposure is proven to be harmful.[34]

These examples provide us with solid evidence which clearly substantiates that the foundation upon which the nation's safety standards are based is deceptive, misleading, and does not protect cell phone users from non-ionizing RF/MW radiation exposure or its associated dangers.

Even though studies have repeatedly shown that deep tissue heating from non-ionizing radiation can cause severe internal tissue damage, destruction of cells, and other adverse health effects without raising bodily temperature, the cellular industry would prefer you to believe that the previously cited notion is true. They are not interested in having you understand how safety standards have been conceived and how absurd they really are; instead they are banking on your trust and ignorance.

The Power of Cell Phone Radiation

RF/MW energy used to transmit communication signals to and from cell phones is extremely powerful. It has the ability to pass through just about any type of matter. When placing a call from wherever you are to whomever you're calling, your signal invariably has to travel through a multitude of objects. To make the connection, invisible microwaves infiltrate metal, glass, concrete, steel, and other seemingly non-penetrable elements. So it's not a stretch to acknowledge the fact that microwaves can just as easily penetrate skin, fat, tissue, and bone. Studies show that when handsets are held against the head, the RF/MW radiation emitted from them delves 2.0 to 3.8 cm (1.5 inches) deep into brain tissue, where it is absorbed and

---

[34] Melbourne, Alan, *"Radiation Protection Standard for Maximum Exposure Levels to Radiofrequency Fields – 3kHz to 300GHz,"* Chapter 4, p.5, http://www.aph.gov.au/SENATE/committee/ecita_ctte/completed_inquiries/1999-02/emr/report/c04.pdf , (March 20, 2002). U.S. exposure guidelines are similarly based.

efficiently heats to cook, damaging and destroying brain cells with every use.[35]

To my knowledge, there are only two exceptions to this rule of penetration. RF/MW signals such as those discharged from cell phones, towers, satellites, and the like are unable to penetrate lead or mountains. This is why you have undoubtedly experienced dropped calls while passing through mountain ranges or driving through hills.

This brings up another interesting point to ponder. When calls are being placed and received by those around you, the waves may actually have to travel through you in order to make the connection. Like second hand smoke, second hand RF/MW radiation exposure from cell phones cannot be contained by the user. Everyone in close proximity of the operator is involuntarily being irradiated, as microwaves pass through everything in their path to link the caller to the receiver. Exposure from other nearby wireless sources, such as Wi-Fi, cell towers, radar, and satellites, also poses serious health concerns.

Dangers resulting from these radiation-emitting apparatuses will be discussed in chapter 10 entitled, Tower Trauma.

Cranial Radiation Absorption

A well-respected group of scientists, working independently of each other, reached a similar conclusion about cell phone radiation absorption. Each reported that as much as 90% of the RF radiation emitted from cell phones is absorbed into the head of the user, instead of dissipating into the atmosphere.[36] There are four key elements that determine actual absorption rates. These include the phone's design, the antenna type, the way in which the phone is used, and the distance the user is from the nearest base station or cell tower.

Your phone's design plays a significant role in the amount of radiation that is absorbed into your head. Every phone has a SAR value that defines the phone's specific absorption rate (SAR). Phones manufactured with a lower SAR factor are supposedly safer than

---

[35] Polk, C., and Postow, E., *CRC Handbook of Biological Effects of Electromagnetic Fields* (Boca Raton, FL: CRC Press, 1986).
[36] Kuster, N., "Multiple Method for Simulating EM Problems Involving Biological Bodies," *IEEE Transactions on Biomedical Engineering* vol. 40, no.7 (July 1993), pp. 611-620.

those with higher SARs. SAR values will be adequately addressed in the upcoming chapter.

The antenna is the most dangerous part of your cell phone, because this is where microwave signals are transmitted to and from. Newer phones with built-in antennas are more dangerous than the older models, which were equipped with retractable antennas. Reason being is that built-in antennas cannot be pulled away from the head to reduce exposure. Instead, these more modern phones emit concentrated amounts of energy, not only from the antenna, but from the entire phone as well.

The way in which you use your phone also determines the amount of radiation that is absorbed into your head. Know that exposure and absorption can be reduced by keeping calls short; limiting the number of calls; holding the phone away from your head while connections are being made; using the speaker feature whenever possible; opting for text messaging or e-mailing; and employing the use of an air headset or another radiation-reducing device. By initiating any one or more of these techniques, you're sure to be better off in the long run.

Chapter 12, entitled Playing it Smart, discusses additional exposure-reducing recommendations.

Lastly, the distance between you and the nearest base station or cell tower also establishes your level of exposure and radiation absorption. The farther away you are from the nearest cell tower, the harder your phone has to work to make a connection. In other words, distance increases the phone's power, thus intensifying your rate of exposure. So, prior to making a call, especially if you're in a remote area, check your phone's signal strength. Signal strength is represented by the number of bars on your phone's screen. Weak signals indicate that you're far away from your service provider's nearest cell site. In these instances, before making or taking a call, it's best to wait for ample signal strength. This will help reduce unnecessary exposure.

The scientific truth that lies behind the distinctiveness of non-ionizing radiation, along with an understanding of deep tissue heating and absorption, can be difficult to grasp. After all, microwaves are invisible and there is no evidence of heat, pain, or discomfort while using your cell phone. What makes this concept even more deceiving is that the brain has no pain receptors. Therefore, even while it's cooking it elicits no warning signs of danger. And without any unpleasant sensations or proof of harm, these issues make the facts look fake, thus misleading you into the illusion that cell phones are safe. The industry has it made in this regard. But please do yourself a favor and keep reading. You'll soon have evidence.

CHAPTER 4

Who's Protecting You?

With over 255 million cell phone users in the U.S, it's baffling that we as a nation remain unaware of the real dangers which have been linked to cell phone radiation exposure. Although a large percentage of cell phone users perceive some level of risk, most are convinced the devices are safe for the casual user. However, the definition of a casual user is constantly being redefined with usage increases. It is also assumed that reasonable government protection is in place.

Emission standard guidelines are parameters that have been established to protect the public from harmful microwave radiation exposure from all wireless communication signals. They are supposed to be set at a level whereby no adverse biological health effects are observed. Unfortunately, as you read through this chapter it will become evident that such objectives have not been met. The terms: 'safety standards', 'emission standards', 'exposure guidelines' and 'safety guidelines' are often used interchangeably to suggest recommended exposure limitations.

With exception of the U.K., the U.S. has the most liberal RF radiation exposure guidelines in the world.[37] In fact, U.S. radiation exposure levels are so high they have been found to be detrimental to the human body. Other countries, such as Sweden, Canada, Eastern Europe, and the former USSR, have restricted their allowable

---

[37] *Doesn't the FCC Standard Protect Us?,*
http://www.goodhealthinfo.net/radiation/fcc_standard.htm (June 2007).

radiation exposure limits by as much as 1,000 times less than those set in the U.S.[38]

You may be wondering why there is such an international discrepancy. Why are Americans permitted to be exposed to so much more radiation than citizens of other countries? After all, don't all human beings have virtually the same biological makeup and aren't all wireless communication signals the same? Wouldn't everybody on the planet be affected in essentially the same manner? The answer is yes.

For years the World Health Organization (WHO) has been trying to adopt a worldwide safety exposure guideline and it has been a definite challenge, since there is such a vast inconsistency in current guidelines among countries. While some countries like the U.K. and the U.S. only recognize dangers at higher exposure levels, other countries are fully aware that dangers exist well below those levels. Since the U.K. and the U.S. have their standards set so high, for reasons you will soon understand, they refuse to reduce their exposure limits to comply with what the rest of the world considers safe. By contrast, countries that are familiar with the development of health hazards at lower exposure levels refuse to raise their limits to comply. They are unwilling to compromise and risk exposing their citizens to what they consider to be perilous conditions.

How Safety Standards Are Established

The chief methods used to determine safety standards of RF/MW radiation exposure in the U.S., as well as internationally, are deceptive. The information on ionizing and non-ionizing radiation provided in the previous chapter should assist you in understanding how U.S. safety standards come into existence.

National and international safety exposure guidelines are founded on five chief components: heating, absorption, short-term research, ignoring studies, and adverse health effects, none of which hold much validity.

---

[38] Robert Kane, *Cellular Telephone Russian Roulette* (New York, NY: Vantage Press, 2001), p. 119.

The dynamics and the effects of thermal radiation exposure in comparison to non-thermal radiation exposure are poles apart. However, the industry, government, and standard setters want you to believe that if, while using your cell phone, there is no sense of heating, then no harm will result. This "No Heat - No Problem" philosophy is extremely misleading; it's a deception, a flat out lie. The rationale behind it is widely accepted as the basis upon which to determine health effects and it is scientifically inept. All wireless communication operations use non-thermal RF/MW radiation. Therefore, setting exposure guidelines solely based on the premise of a heating and thermal response is absurd.

The standards which have been set in place for your protection are first and foremost devised to protect you from immediate, external thermal dangers, such as burns; this response from non-thermal microwave radiation exposure is highly unlikely. However, depending on its intensity, non-ionizing microwave radiation can generate a deep tissue heating response well below the skin's surface without ever being detected. If the body is able to compensate for and dissipate the heat load, there is little reason to believe that damage will take place. But if heating cannot be compensated for or previous damage is irreparable, further damage will result and possibly compound.[39]

Even as standard setters work to convince you that no harm exists without heating, it is important to recognize that very significant adverse health effects have been observed at non-thermal levels. Many even transpire at exposure levels far below the current safety guidelines and occur prior to any tissue heating. The non-thermal radiation exposure you are inundated with everyday, from cell phones and other radiation-emitting devices, have been found to produce a variety of biological and neurological effects. Some of these effects include abnormal brain activity; unusual and aggressive behavior; mood swings, reduced learning ability and performance; sleep disturbances; reproductive consequences; cancer; DNA damage; reduced immunity; hormonal changes; and cell proliferation. Therefore, a safety standard that only considers the heating effects of non-ionizing radiation is unrealistic...and irresponsible.

---

[39] Brown, Gary, *Wireless Devices, Standards, and Microwave Radiation in the Education Environment*, http://www.emfacts.com/wlans.html (October 2000).

Absorption

Safety standards are also founded on the assumption that the human body absorbs RF/MW radiation equally, but research indicates otherwise. Cell phone radiation does not irradiate the human body evenly; neither is it absorbed uniformly. If these statements were true, this criterion would make sense. But the truth of the matter is that some tissue has been shown to be more vulnerable than other tissue. Brain tissue, for instance, is extremely sensitive to high rates of RF/MW radiation absorption. Scientific researchers N. Kuster, O. Gandhi, G. Lovisolo, and V. Hombach all specialize in this field and agree that between 50% to 90%+ of the RF/MW radiation emitted from cell phones is deposited into and absorbed by the user's brain.[40] Eyes and breasts are also particularly responsive to this radiant energy. [41] Some organs and tissue located near the waist are likewise posed with an elevated risk of danger. The kidneys, the liver, and the testes absorb radiation more readily than other mid to lower range body parts.

An informational pamphlet accompanying every Verizon cell phone affirms this very point by stating that, "if the phone is mounted against the waist or other part of the body (head) during use (or while it's "on"), then that part of the body will absorb more RF energy."

Exposure guidelines also conclude that the human body can safely absorb up to 5 W/kg (watts per kilogram) of radiation before there is an internal temperature increase of 1° C (1.9° Fahrenheit). It is wrongly assumed that temperature increases below this level, cause no health problems.

To clarify this unrealistic concept, bear in mind the example given in the last chapter concerning whole body heating, tissue absorption, and distribution. Adverse health effects like pain and a burning sensation transpire after holding your finger over a candle flame for an extended period of time. But continued exposure will never be evenly distributed throughout the body, nor will it heat the entire body enough to produce an internal temperature increase of 1° C. This demonstrates how some forms of heat, including that of non-

---

[40] Robert Kane, *Cellular Telephone Russian Roulette* (New York, NY: Vantage Press, 2001), p. 8.
[41] Begich, Nick and Roderick, James, *Earthpulse Press, Inc.*, "Cell Phone Convenience or 21st Century Plague?,"
http://www.earthpulse.com/products/cellphoneplague.htm (July 2004).

ionizing microwave radiation, are not evenly absorbed or distributed, but do still cause damage.

Different parts of the body respond differently to various doses of radiation exposure. This further demonstrates how concentrated amounts of RF/MW radiation aimed at particular bodily areas, like those previously mentioned, can significantly impact the tissue in those areas without affecting the rest of the body. The misconception that this type of radiation is equally absorbed and distributed also provides insight as to how inadequate, deceptive, and misleading the foundation upon which our so-called safety standards are based.

Short Term Research

Not only are national exposure guidelines established on the immediate hazards associated with heating, equal absorption and distribution of radiation, but the underlying data used to determine safety is derived solely from short-term exposure studies. Standard setters do not take into consideration the adverse health effects which have been shown to occur from long-term exposure to non-thermal RF/MW radiation, like those which can result after years of cell phone use.

Although multiple short-term research efforts have revealed and confirmed adverse health effects, very few people experience short-term exposure. Since RF/MW radiation is not limited to cell phone use, even those without the communication device are being irradiated with exposure from cell towers and other forms of wireless communication, such as Wi-Fi, cordless phones, satellite, and radar. Chronic exposure to this harmful energy invades the daily life of most people. It's just that the near-range exposure of radiant energy that is aimed directly into your head via your cell phone is more concentrated and more dangerous, because the human body is less able to compensate for such a close-range assault.

Ignoring Potentially Damaging Studies

In 1995, Dr. Ross Adey, a world renowned senior research expert in this area and a widely published RF researcher from the University of California, Riverside commented, "The laboratory evidence for a-thermal effects of both ELF (extra low frequency) and RF/Microwave fields now constitutes a major body of scientific literature in peer-reviewed journals (which scientists and attorneys rely on for proof of evidence). It is my personal view that to continue to ignore this work in the course of standard setting is irresponsible to the point of being a public scandal." "It is 'not a level playing field' in rejecting the evidence, in many cases peer reviewed and published, for non-thermal effects while uncritically accepting very questionable studies and claiming no effects were found. You can't have it both ways!" [42]

But instead of reviewing all of the available data and looking at the issue objectively, the FCC elected to side with industry interests, choosing which studies to consider and which ones to ignore.[43] Such an important decision regarding American's safety should be established only after conducting a thorough examination of all credible research and studies, not just a select few or those funded by the industry where the outcomes can be and often are pre-determined.

In 1999 the federal Radiofrequency Interagency Work Group (RFIAWG) of non-ionizing radiation experts issued a RF Guidelines Statement. RFIAWG is comprised of members in U.S. agencies including the FDA, NIOSH (National Institute for Occupational Safety and Health), EPA, OSHA (Occupational Safety and Health Administration), and NTIA (National Telecommunications and Information Administration). This federal agency group disagreed with the FCC when they maintained that their guidelines protected the public from harmful exposure. As mentioned earlier, there were a number of things that were never taken into account when safety guidelines were set.[44]

---

[42] Maisch, Don, *"Submissions to Standards Australia on Adopting the ICNIRP Radio Frequency Exposure Limits for Australia and New Zealand"*. "ICNIRP RF/MW Guidelines for Australia / New Zealand" Discussion paper (A), July 24, 1998.

[43] Robert Kane, *Cellular Telephone Russian Roulette* (New York, NY: Vantage Press, 2001), p. 141.

[44] Brown, Gary, *Wireless Devices, Standards, and Microwave Radiation in the Education Environment,* http://www.emfacts.com/wlans.html (October 2000).

In September 1999, theoretical physicist Dr. Gerard Hyland wrote the following in an appendix to the Minutes of Evidence, which was addressed to the British Parliament's Select Committee on Science and Technology: "Although the existing safety guidelines are clearly necessary, they are quite inadequate. For they completely fail to consider the possibility of adverse health effects linked to the fact that living organisms – and only living ones – have the ability to respond to aspects of technologically produced radiation other than its intensity, and, accordingly, can respond at intensities well below the limits imposed by the safety guidelines." [45]

While this statement was made regarding standards established in the U.K., the premise upon which it stands equally applies to the course of action taken in the U.S. The human body is electrical and it operates on electrical impulses, impulses which are influenced and affected by RF/MW signals. This external interference causes internal problems.

In the U.S., a number of animal laboratory studies were conducted in order to determine where safety standards for humans should be established. Researchers sought to find the lowest RF/MW radiation exposure levels that would elicit adverse behavioral effects and, since safety was presumably the ultimate goal, limits would have logically been set prior to observing *any* change in behavior.

However, instead of following logical criteria, industry scientists often waited until an animal's activity level dropped as low as 67% before recording any behavioral change (adverse effect). If standard setters were really interested in establishing safe public exposure limits, why would they wait until research subjects experienced such a significant decline in performance? Consider how even a 50% drop in your daily performance and ability would affect your job, your relationships, your lifestyle, and your overall quality of life. You would likely not be able to do half as much as you usually do and you'd probably only be able to do it half as well.

Clearly, each one of the five components upon which safety standards are based - heating, absorption, short-term research, ignoring studies, and adverse health effects - warrant delusions of protection. Rather than aggressively pursuing safety for American

---

[45] Petition for Inquiry of the EMR Network, Before the Federal Communications Commission, September 25, 2001, presented by attorney James R. Hobson, Miller & Van Eaton, P.L.L.C., Washington, D.C.

citizens, the FCC, along with standard setters, are knowingly and willfully allowing you to be exposed to levels of radiation that have been proven to alter behavior and cause harm. Guidelines based on false pretenses, such as those previously mentioned, continue to deceive the public into believing that cell phones are safe.

The rise in public health concerns, along with proof of non-thermal adverse health effects occurring at levels well below those which are considered safe, suggests that the government should make more of an effort to budget money for independent research. But since allocating funds to ensure public safety still hasn't happened in the U.S., some Americans might tend to believe what Norm Alster, writer for *Investor's Business Daily*, stated a decade ago: "With the government depending on revenue from operating wireless carriers, Washington is telling the public 'your health concerns don't count.'" [46]

Who Sets Safety Standards?

Who are the people setting these safety standards? Who do you rely on to keep you safe? Who are you trusting to make such important decisions on your behalf?

Most would consider it reasonable to assume that the people making health-related determinations about how radiant energy affects the human body are medical professionals or public health officials. But this is not the case.

Standard guidelines for public safety and exposure limits to RF/MW radiation emitted from wireless devices and their sites are not established by government agencies. Neither do those who hold any kind of medical or health-related degree determine them. Rather than recruiting knowledgeable, unbiased third-party individuals to design safety criteria on behalf of American citizens, the U.S. Government relies on three scientific organizations: the Institute of Electrical and Electronic Engineers (IEEE or "I-triple E"), the American National Standards Institute (ANSI or "an-see"), and the National Council on Radiation Protection and Measurements (NCRP). These organizations are responsible for issuing national guidelines, often referred to as the ANSI/IEEE standards, for adoption by the FCC. These guidelines set conforming parameters for the industry.

---

[46] Alster, Norm, "Newspaper Questions Whether Government has Considered 'Risks' of Wireless", *Investor's Business Daily*, May 29, 1997.

Since 1982, the ANSI and the IEEE have been the principal sources of expert advice to the FCC, regarding RFR (radiofrequency radiation), RF/MW exposure, and its related hazards.[47] The ANSI sets criterion standards for a multitude of unrelated electronic devices and the IEEE specializes in wireless technology.

The IEEE is a professional association made up of electronic engineers and physicists who are most familiar with the characteristics of radiation. Members of the IEEE have very close ties with the cell phone industry and the military. Is a matter of fact, an article published in *Microwave News*, a trusted trade journal which reports on industry happenings, disclosed that, "Standard setting bodies do more or less as the industry wants. Their members are often current, past, or future employees of the very companies they are supposed to regulate. Meanwhile government agencies have no appetite for confrontation".[48]

And although it's apparent that the IEEE standard setting committee is comprised of experts who know how to make wireless technology work, they are not experts in understanding how its radiation interacts with and affects the human body. A 2001 *Microwave News* editorial recognized this problem stating, "The Pentagon's new microwave weapon has been brought to you by...the same organizations that control the IEEE's SCC-28 committee that writes the standard for exposures to RF and microwaves....It seems obvious, yet worth repeating...Health standards should be written by medical and public health professionals, not those who make weapons for the military-industrial complex."[49]

Upon realizing that national standards are not prescribed by medical or healthcare professionals, but by scientists, engineers, and physicists who have ulterior motives which coincide with the industry, you are likely to agree with insider Dr. Robert Kane's assessment. In his book, *Cellular Telephone Russian Roulette*, Kane warns the public to be particularly wary of those who make the rules and decisions regarding safety in this country, because they are economically interested parties who are bias in their opinions and

---

[47] Petition for Inquiry of the EMR Network, Before the Federal Communications Commission, September 25, 2001, presented by attorney James R. Hobson, Miller & Van Eaton, P.L.L.C., Washington, D.C.
[48] Brown, Gary, *Wireless Devices, Standards, and Microwave Radiation in the Education Environment,* http://www.emfacts.com/wlans.html (October 2000).
[49] *Doesn't the FCC Standard Protect Us?,*
http://www.goodhealthinfo.net/radiation/fcc_standard.htm (June 2007).

who are "acting in concert with your government." "Make no mistake, the success of the cellular telephone industry is significant revenue business for the government."

Therefore, instead of setting limits well below those which are known to cause multiple adverse health effects, the determination seems to be that the nation is willing to assume an "acceptable risk." The only problem with this assumption is that full disclosure of the risks assumed is not forthcoming.[50]

Cell Phone Regulation or Exemption?

If you still believe that somehow you are being protected from harmful cell phone radiation exposure, after reading this section you might believe otherwise.

Prior to 1993, there was no scientific evidence of thermal adverse health effects from radio waves below 40 W/kg, so it appeared that cell phones operating on less than 1 W/kg were no threat. Based on that premise alone, FDA scientists and government officials exempted cell phones from having to comply with the IEEE/ANSI safety exposure guidelines. Cell phones were also immune from having to meet any type of regulatory standard and were excused from all government mandated pre-market testing obligations.[51]

These decisions were wrongly substantiated, based exclusively on the thermal effects of radiation. The thermal effects, which result from the non-ionizing radiation of cell phones, were never even taken into account. As a result, the cell phone industry has been granted an undeserved and uncontrolled freedom that is just as economically satisfying for the industry as it is for standard setters and the government.

Dr. Quirino Balzano, a top Motorola scientist, confirms the exemption that the industry has been unjustifiably granted by saying: "With the current budget cut-backs, the agencies of the government will not have the time, the funds and the personnel to research the particular exposure conditions of the mobile communications transmitters. It is up to the industry to show reasonable evidence of adherence to safety standards and receive categorical exclusions."

---

[50] Robert Kane, *Cellular Telephone Russian Roulette* (New York, NY: Vantage Press, 2001), p. 116.
[51] George Carlo and Martin Schram, *Cell Phones: Invisible Hazards of the Wireless Age* (New York, NY: Carroll & Graf Publishers, 2001), p. 21.

Balzano further depicts the industry's primary concern with regard to complying with set safety standards: "Their proposition is that, since they don't quite understand the physics relating to electromagnetic fields to the near-zone of antennas, safety standards should not be enforced because it would be detrimental to the industry. Stricter safety guidelines will lead to increased legal problems."

To add to the perplexity, Dr. Kane quotes R. Cleveland, a FCC representative, as making the following startling confession during a private conversation: "The FCC doesn't want to regulate portable cellular telephones because it doesn't want to create a panic."[52]

It is not surprising that the exemption was fully agreed upon and accepted by the IEEE, the ANSI, and the FCC standard setting committees, as well as the cell phone industry. The decision to make cell phones exempt took place in much the same way as it did with the tobacco industry exemption. Tobacco products were successfully freed from having to comply with certain agricultural, environmental, and drug regulations which would have rendered them unsafe. As it was with the tobacco industry, lobbyists and cell phone industry representatives have triumphantly convinced the government to grant them unrealistic proposals of exemption, at the public's expense.

Kane makes two profound observations about this mind-boggling cell phone immunity. First, he claims that, "if it were not for the exemption that the industry promoted, the portables would be in violation of all accepted safety standards now in existence." And second, that, "if it were not for the categorical exclusion that exempted portable cellular telephones from any radiation exposure regulations, the devices would have been barred from the marketplace as unsafe for humans!"[53]

Apparently, the reason cell phones were exempt up to 1996 and safety standards concerning them were not being enforced is, as Balzano stated, because it would have been greatly detrimental to the industry. If cell phone power was reduced, they could be deemed useless and, if cell phones had to comply with what seem to be restrictive safety guidelines, the invitation for lawsuits would be extensive.

---

[52] Robert Kane, *Cellular Telephone Russian Roulette* (New York, NY: Vantage Press, 2001), pp. 122-123, 141.
[53] Ibid. pp. 10, 117-118, 195.

Therefore, rather than the government mandating safety and forcing the industry to take all necessary precautions to protect consumers, it granted the industry an exemption which allowed them to bypass all established safety measures. Outside of financial gain, it is difficult to understand why the needs of the wireless industry supersede those of the American people.

Specific Absorption Rate (SAR)

Today, there is one criterion that the industry is supposed to adhere to regarding cell phones; they are to limit cell phone exposure to specific absorption rate (SAR) parameters. SAR is a complex method of measurement used to determine radiation exposure and it represents the relative absorption of energy per second (watts), per unit of body mass (kilograms) at any given time. It is referred to as "watts per kilogram" and is written W/kg.[54] Two elements - frequency and power - are used to determine SAR. Varying frequency levels and power densities (energy + distance) result in different rates of absorption.

On the surface SAR measurements may seem practical and sound like valid preventative assurances, but these computations continue to be based on the assumption that all human tissue absorbs radiation at the same rate and that radiation is equally distributed. SAR averages radiation absorption taken from any one cubic gram of tissue, at any given time, rather than identifying organs such as the brain, which readily absorbs RF/MW radiation at a faster pace and is much more vulnerable to its intrusive energy.

Additionally, the SAR method of measurement is deceiving, because it can easily be manipulated to serve a given purpose. For example, averaging an SAR of 2 W/kg over 10 grams of tissue has an SAR of up to 6 W/kg when averaged over 1 gram of tissue. In other words, SAR can be significantly reduced by averaging absorption rates over a larger body mass. Due to this variance, it becomes readily apparent that cell phone users can be exposed to higher radiation levels than those allowed by SAR standards, without knowledge or consent.[55]

---

[54] Petition for Inquiry of the EMR Network, Before the Federal Communications Commission, September 25, 2001, presented by attorney James R. Hobson, Miller & Van Eaton, P.L.L.C., Washington, D.C.

[55] Melbourne, Alan, *Problems with the Rationale of the Draft Standard,* http://www.ssec.org.au/emraa/rf/may.htm (May 11, 2001).

Current IEEE/ANSI exposure guidelines for cell phones are set at an SAR of 1.6 W/kg. Some may assume that this level of exposure is extremely low and must offer some element of safety, but Dr. Henry Lai, one of the top biophysicist's in the field, disagrees. He, along with other researchers, have ascertained that biological consequences, such as cellular DNA damage, increased calcium efflux in cells, and decreased cell division, all transpire at exposure levels as low as 0.001 W/kg.[56] Although these small numbers may not seem like much, there is a huge difference between 1.6 W/kg and 0.001 W/kg. 1.6 W/kg is 1600 times greater than 0.001 W/kg.

The Environmental Protection Agency (EPA) also expressed concern, recognizing an SAR of 1.6 W/kg as being an unacceptable and unrealistic level of exposure to ensure safety. The agency reported, "The data currently available on the relationship of SAR to biological effects show evidence for biological affects at an SAR of about 1 W/kg." "In view of these laboratory studies, there is reason to believe that the findings of carcinogenicity in humans are biologically plausible."[57] Nevertheless, this is the safety guideline which has been adopted by the FCC.

Since the FCC lacks the necessary manpower and funding to ensure compliance, they fully rely on the self-regulated industry to conduct their own testing. To assess the reliability and adherence of cell phone manufacturers complying with prescribed SAR exposure limits, some phones were put to the test on ABC's 20/20 news program. Multiple testing methods were employed and the results were closely observed. It was discovered that several brands of cell phones exceeded the already detrimental national radiation exposure limit.[58]

If the RF/MW energy emitted from cell phones was evenly dispersed and absorbed throughout the entire body, SAR measurements might make more sense. If adverse non-thermal effects were taken into account, rather than ignored, SAR standards might be more satisfactory. If testing requirements were more

---

[56] Kasevich, Raymond S., *CS Medical Technologies LLC,* "Cell phones, Radar, and Health", http://www.spectrum.ieee.org/WEBONLY/resource/aug02/speak2.html (2006)

[57] Robert Kane, *Cellular Telephone Russian Roulette* (New York, NY: Vantage Press, 2001), p. 83.

[58] Begich, Nick and Roderick, James, *Earthpulse Press, Inc.,* "Cell Phone Convenience or 21st Century Plague?,"
http://www.earthpulse.com/products/cellphoneplague.htm (July 2004).

stringent for manufacturers and an objective third-party was responsible for assuring compliance, the American people could have more confidence in these SAR exposure guidelines. And, most importantly, if standards that prevented any and all adverse health effects from occurring were accepted, the public could take comfort in being adequately protected. But the fact remains, SAR standards are clearly a deceptive way of falsely insuring safety.

CHAPTER 5

No Health Risks?

If cell phones pose no adverse health risks, then why have the FDA and the EPA made the following recommendations to consumers: limit cell phone use to emergency situations; reduce unnecessary calls; and use landline phones whenever possible?[59]

It's also peculiar that in October 2002, over one hundred German doctors signed a petition, stating that increased health problems resulting from cell phone use and chronic cell tower exposure were on the rise and being observed in numerous patients.[60] These medical professionals are not alone in their observations. Governments, organizations, scientists, researchers, and experts from around the world have also recognized a comparable impact and have expressed similar concern.

If you are a cell phone user who is unwilling to accept that any health risks, other then rare cases of brain cancer or brain tumors, have been linked to RF/MW radiation exposure, this chapter will give you much to consider. If nothing more, it should challenge you to contemplate whether cell phones are as safe as the industry has led you to believe.

---

[59] Robert Kane, *Cellular Telephone Russian Roulette* (New York, NY: Vantage Press, 2001), p. 229.
[60] The Freiburger Appeal. http://www.emrnetwork.org/news/IGUMED_english.pdf (October 2002).

If there are no health risks tied to cell phone use and cell tower emissions, then why were U.S. pharmaceutical companies so eager to dump millions of dollars into the research and development of new drugs that would alleviate the exact symptoms that have been linked to RF/MW radiation exposure?

Personally, I don't believe in coincidences, especially in situations like these. Big businesses are shrewd and they usually only fork out hefty sums of money when they are all but guaranteed that their investment will produce an extremely lucrative return. Instead, I am led to presume that there was more than enough foreknowledge and scientific evidence for the pharmaceutical industry to invest in the upcoming needs of those who would suffer from RF/MW radiation exposure.

Studies focusing on this topic and revealing the body's undesirable response began decades prior to the emergence of cell phones. For example, in the early 1950s, the U.S. government was naive and reluctant to acknowledge that dangers existed from non-ionizing radiation exposure. To test their theory and to prove a point, in 1953 the Russians began irradiating the U.S. embassy in Moscow with low power microwaves, like those used to transmit cell phone signals. This invisible assault went on for close to 19 years, continuing long after the U.S. government was notified as to what was happening and who was responsible.

Yet, even after the discovery of the "Moscow signal" in 1962, the government allowed the experimental conduct to persist for another 10 years. The embassy staff was completely unaware that they were being involuntarily and chronically bombarded with RF/MW radiation. Instead of looking out for its employee's best interests, the U.S. government chose to use them as guinea pigs to test the relevance of the Russians' theory that non-ionizing microwaves were harmful to the human body. Furthermore, in order to properly examine and evaluate the situation, the CIA (Central Intelligence Agency) requested the assistance of an expert in the field to help decipher the ongoing data.

After close analysis of the information gathered from U.S. embassy staff, numerous symptoms were identified as being characteristic responses to this type of exposure. There was no question that a direct link existed between health complaints, measurable disorders, and the invisible, undetected RF/MW exposure they were all irradiated with. The commonalties of headache, fatigue, anxiety, dizziness, insomnia, concentration difficulties, memory loss, depression and more, have since been confirmed time and time again in multiple research efforts. The consistent development of these seemingly unrelated exposure-induced ailments has led to a debilitating disease which has been appropriately labeled Microwave Sickness.[61]

Ironically, after learning that consumers were going to be faced with this chronic source of exposure, the pharmaceutical industry got busy developing and manufacturing drugs to help alleviate every symptom which corresponded to those of Microwave Sickness. Western doctors, who remain uninformed of this global syndrome, continue to advocate the various drugs emerging from the pharmaceutical industry. The majority are clueless as to the source of aggravation, treating each symptom as if it was unrelated to the others.

Again, it's hard to believe that the development of said drugs was purely coincidental; that the pharmaceutical industry was acting solely on hunches when they began creating drugs that miraculously addressed every single exposure-induced symptom. However, pharmaceutical companies weren't the only ones able to capitalize on a fore knowledge of the effects of non-ionizing microwave radiation. The medical industry also discovered how to utilize the same technology to their advantage.

Medical Use of Non-ionizing Microwave Radiation

If cell phone microwaves are not biologically reactive, then it's curious to understand why the medical community is rapidly incorporating the use of non-ionizing microwave radiation into numerous medical procedures. Such procedures include those which successfully heat and destroy deep bodily tissue, utilizing the same low power and frequencies as cell phones.

From as far back as 50 years, research findings have shown that electromagnetic waves induce effective and efficient deep tissue heating to the area in which its rays are directed.[62] To this day,

---

[61] Becker, Robert, O. and Selden, Gary, *The Body Electric* (New York, NY: William Morrow and Company, Inc., 1985), pp. 314-315.

[62] Schwan, H., P., and Piersol, G., M., "The Absorption of Electromagnetic Energy in Body Tissues," *International Review of Physical Medicine and Rehabilitation,* June 1955, pp. 424-448.

radiant therapy continues to successfully heal bone fractures and deep tissue wounds. Applications are also used in post surgical procedures to speed healing by reducing pain and swelling.

The low intensity EMFs (electromagnetic fields) that interact with the body so efficiently for medical purposes are at exposure levels well below current safety standards. This means that, while you are being told that no biological effects occur from the same type of exposure, there are medical applications being implemented that prove otherwise. The irony here is that the FDA approves of medically related radiation treatment devices, because it recognizes the body's positive response to them. Yet, when it comes to cell phone and cell tower exposure, it denies that the same category of low power signals has the potential to adversely interact with the human body.[63]

Even more unsettling, is the fact that medical professionals have determined that the 700-1000 MHz range of RF/MW radiation interacts most effectively with human tissue. Of this frequency range, it's believed that waves between 750-900 MHz are best suited for deep tissue penetration, cell destruction, as well as heating and radiation absorption without initiating pain. This same medically-preferred frequency range is also best for cell phone operation. Because of their distinctive properties, these frequencies are also the most dangerous frequencies known to man!

One such medical treatment that successfully implements this source of energy is diathermy. During this treatment non-ionizing radiation is used to heat tissue below the skin's surface, without the patient experiencing any pain or discomfort. Although diathermy treatments must heat tissue in order to be effective, it does not desire to cause damage. However, this is difficult to avoid. As with cell phone use, the rays used in diathermy treatments are delivered at 900 MHz in order to achieve deep tissue heating. Experiments with this treatment show that the characteristics of the two scenarios – diathermy and consumer cell phone use - are "so similar as to be indistinguishable."

Hyperthermia, another medical treatment, is a cancer radiation therapy technique used to destroy cancerous cells via deep tissue heating. Here in the U. S., it has been discovered that non-ionizing frequencies between 700-950 MHz can effortlessly attain this goal. Non-thermal microwave radiation targets cancerous cells,

---

[63] Sage, C., *The Bio Initiative Report*,
http://www.bioinitiative.org/report/docs/section_1.pdf (May 2008), p. 20

purposely intending to destroy them, but unfortunately what happens is that healthy cells are annihilated along with the cancerous ones. Since cells are in such close proximity, they can't be differentiated. This technique is very efficient and can be initiated without pain, burning sensations or discomfort.[64]

Similarly, in 2003, the U.K. government, along with the National Institute of Clinical Excellence (NICE), approved what has come to be referred to as "The 3-Minute Hysterectomy." This treatment is performed using a hand-held wand that removes the lining of the womb quickly and easily by emitting low-powered microwaves. The microwave emissions from the 'wand' heat and destroy uterine wall tissue without eliciting any pain, scarring or burning.[65]

These examples firmly reinforce just how inadequate and absurd U.S. safety standards are, by suggesting that without an internal rise in temperature no damage or adverse effects can occur.

Radiation procedures for multiple medical applications are being employed where the destruction of deep tissue is necessary to obtain the desired outcome. Realizing the powerful potential of microwaves, one has to wonder: If cell phones expose users to the same kind of non-ionizing frequencies of low power used in these medical procedures, how can holding a cell phone up to one's head *not* be harmful?

Military Use of Non-lethal Weapons

Last I knew, weapons were meant to inflict harm and to destroy an enemy. Although highly classified, the fact of the matter is that, for the past 40 years, electromagnetic, RF, and microwave technology at intensified levels, has been used to develop weapons that emit energy signals. These types of weapons are now being incorporated into the military armories of numerous countries around the world.[66] According to the former head of the Defense Intelligence Agency (DIA), Leonard Perroots, "the advent into the world's arsenals of directed energy weapons may be as revolutionary

---

[64] Robert Kane, *Cellular Telephone Russian Roulette* (New York, NY: Vantage Press, 2001), pp. 18-19, 22, 52, 202.

[65] "Energy Medicine/Positive Proof of MW-bio-effects", *Citizens' Initiative Omega*, October 7, 2003.

[66] Welsh, Cheryl, *Non-lethal Weapons, A Global Issue*, http://www.raven1.net/welshnlw.htm (November 2001).

as was the introduction of the other great weapon developments of the 20th century - the machine-gun and the atomic bomb." U.S. experts say that the Soviet Union has the edge over the United States in developing what is known as "directed energy weapons" and "radiofrequency weapons."[67]

Radiofrequency electromagnetic weapons are considered non-lethal, because, even though their rays have the capacity to kill, they are not devised for that purpose. Instead, they are developed to inflict an unfamiliar form of torture and manipulation. This type of energy can easily disable computers, interfere with other wireless signals, and intervene with sensitive equipment, and in military combat this can be extremely advantageous.

However, pulses from these non-lethal weapons can do so much more. Signals can target the brain to interfere with normal, natural functioning and generate programmed responses. They can manipulate brain waves and cause subjects, both animal and human, to fall into a stupor, to experience flu-like symptoms, to become nauseated, to sleep or stay awake, and even to become confused and disorientated. Wave frequency can also match brain activity to control the victim's mind and manipulate the human psyche.

Like other weapons of warfare, these extremely powerful signals can be directed into groups. Whether the goal is to irradiate one person or many people, the waves invade without detection. There is never any evidence of an attack; there is no explosion or noise; and rarely is any pain or discomfort experienced. As it was with the irradiation of the U.S. Embassy in Moscow, anyone can be victimized by this silent antagonist and be completely unaware of the assault.

In combat these weapons are multi-functional. "The microwave bomb, which works by emitting a massive pulse of radio energy, would render humans unconscious by scrambling neural paths in the brain, but would not cause lasting injury."[68] The Vice President of the Russian Academy of Military Science, Vladimir Slipchenko, [stated that]: By directing energy emissions at a target it is possible to turn an enemy division into a herd of frightened

[67] Debusmann, Bernard, "Beam Weapons Predicted to Revolutionize War, Spur Arms Trade." Reuter *Library Report BC cycle.* Lexis-Nexis. March 28, 1990.
[68] Campbell, Christy, "Microwave Bomb That Does Not Kill", *Sunday Telegraph,* September 27, 1992, p. 6.

idiots.[69]   Additionally, "[U.S. Air Force Major], Norman Routanen has proposed using very powerful microwave devices to confuse, disable, or even kill the enemy."[70]

RF energy also has a profound impact on breathing. Captain Paul Tyler, director of the U.S. Navy Electromagnetic Radiation Project from 1970-1977, stated: "It has been shown that normal breathing takes place at certain frequencies and amplitudes and not at others. Animals (like humans) forced to breathe at certain unnatural frequencies develop severe respiratory distress." Such difficulties can result in feelings of uneasiness and anxiety, which can lead to suffocation, even resulting in death.[71]

Mind Control

Mind control has also been researched by governments and has been going on since the 1940s. If you've ever had occasion to watch someone be hypnotized, you were likely made aware of how the power of suggestion can be used to render an immediate, delayed, or word-provoked action. The use of RF energy aimed into a person's brain can trigger the same types of responses. Emotions, behaviors, and actions can all be roused without the subject's conscious awareness of what is taking place or why. Also, amnesia-like symptoms can be projected, to inhibit the recall of information, events or situations. Some people willingly seek to be hypnotized to revert to past memories, to quit smoking, or to lose weight, but there are others who are involuntarily and unknowingly being exposed to this same type of mind control.

Dr. William Van Bise, a radio engineer who investigated the 1970s Russian Woodpecker radio signal that was broadcast throughout the U.S., said that the easiest way to disrupt the mental process would be with microwaves. Pulsed microwaves, like those in digital phones, have been successfully used for mind control; they work like subliminal messaging. Inaudible messages can be transferred through microwaves into the subconscious mind, effectively bypassing the conscious, to conveniently change thoughts

---

[69] Pillsbury, Michael, Senate Intelligence Committee. *Federal News Service.* Lexis-Nexis, September 18, 1997.
[70] Miller, Marc S., "Ambiguous War the United States and Low-Intensity Conflict", *MIT Alumni Association Technology Review,* August 1987, Vol. 90 p. 60.
[71] "Have the Radiofrequency Weapons Been Put to Use Yet?," http://www.wealth4freedom.com/truth/12/mindcontrol.htm (November 2002).

and behavior. Signals from outside radiation sources, using electromagnetic technology, can imitate the mind's electrical pulses. Persons under attack are completely unaware that their thoughts, responses, and actions are being influenced by someone other than themselves.[72]

In 1963, Dr. George Estabrooks, the man who initially proposed the use of hypnosis in military warfare, admitted to doing extensive work for the CIA, the FBI, and military intelligence. He referred to his occupation as "child's play," because he was able to successfully create an effective spy, a dedicated assassin, and even change the personalities of unsuspecting subjects. During the same year President Kennedy was shot, Estabrooks suggested that Lee Harvey Oswald and Jack Ruby "could have very well been performing through hypnosis."[73]

Between 1953-1972, when the Russians were irradiating the U.S. embassy in Moscow with non-ionizing microwaves, some curious happenings transpired. For instance, during a Senate hearing on MKULTRA (the CIA's Program of Research into Behavioral Modification) in September 1977, Dr. Gottlieb, director of experiments, warned congress that the Russians had been actively pursuing the use of intelligence weapons against the U.S. Government. Even more curious is that, while traveling to Russia in 1972, President Nixon's staff reported his behavior as being 'inappropriate' at times, recalling instances when he would cry without provocation.[74]

The 1967 mood altering and mind control experiments at Montauk Point, a U.S. Air Force base in New York's Long Island, offer another case in point. It was discovered that, by changing the frequency and pulse duration of the Sage radar, transmission of electromagnetic waves uniformly changed the personality and mood of everyone exposed.

The experiment began on a small scale, yet within a very short period of time military technicians expanded the radar's signal to reach upstate New York, New Jersey, and Connecticut. Using special technology, technicians were able to assemble each irradiated

---

[72] "David Brinkley News Program," #47592, aired July 16, 1981.

[73] Anonymous, *Mind Control and The Intelligence Services*, http://www.wakeupmag.co.uk/articles/mind.htm

[74] Welsh, Cheryl, *U.S. Human Rights Abuse Report: A Factual Report in Support of the need for International Investigation,* http://www.dcn.davis.ca.us/~welsh/7.htm (January 1998).

person's thoughts, and have their computers translate the data and display the results on their screens.[75]

Even now, U.S. Defense has an active project in Alaska, known as H.A.A.R.P. (High-frequency Active Auroral Research Project), which has similar capabilities of administering this type of mind control. An expert reveals that, "HAARP is a secret undertaking that is not unlike the Manhattan Project, which gave us the atomic bomb."[76]

The idea of being able to project one's thoughts into someone else's mind is extremely bizarre, yet it is no longer science fiction.

The purpose for sharing this information with you regarding the use of microwaves as non-lethal weapons is not to insinuate that this type of manipulation and mind control is taking place through the waves being emitted from your cell phone or from cell towers. It is simply to acquaint you with the incredible power and magnificent impact these invisible and undetectable microwave signals have.

Radiation Shielding Patents

If cell phones aren't dangerous, then it's difficult to understand why the leading cell phone manufacturers have spent thousands of dollars over the past 15 years quietly acquiring various radiation shielding patents to protect consumers from their phone's emissions. In the mid-to-late 1990s, Nokia, the number one cell phone supplier, obtained multiple patents to reduce electromagnetic (RF/MW) radiation exposure to cell phone users' heads. Motorola and Ericsson have also received various radiation-reducing patents for their phones. Other radiation-reducing patents have been secured by Hitachi, Mitsubishi, and Alcatel N. V.

"The patents speak for themselves. Here these folks have the ability to protect consumers from being radiated and they're unwilling to spend a couple bucks to do so. It's outrageous," declares attorney Carl Hilliard, wireless safety advocate.[77]

---

[75] Anonymous, *Mind Control and The Intelligence Services,* http://www.wakeupmag.co.uk/articles/mind.htm
[76] Welsh, Cheryl, *U.S. Human Rights Abuse Report: A Factual Report in Support of the need for International Investigation,* http://www.dcn.davis.ca.us/~welsh/7.htm (January 1998).
[77] Silva, Jeffery, "Manufacturers (Nokia's) Own Patents to Cut Radiation", *RCR Wireless News,* June 4, 2001.

Dr. Kane discloses what he learned as an industry insider, "Even while the numerous reports of high energy absorptions continue, manufacturers claim there is no possibility of harm as a result of operating their portable phones. However, it is known that they engaged in research to shield the heads and brains of users from the penetrating radiation – but only after the hazard issue became public."[78]

Long Term Studies Proving Safety

If cell phones aren't dangerous, then why has the industry refused to fund any long term studies to prove safety? In an effort to have them do just that, Dr. Elizabeth Jacobson, the FDA's Director of Science, recommended that the CTIA incorporate critical post-market surveillance studies as "an ongoing cost of doing business". But the recommendation was never taken seriously.

According to Dr. Carlo, in a 1997 meeting with three top Motorola executives, the importance of a post-market plan was brought up, only to be quickly shot down. Another attempt was made to convince those at the CTIA of the necessity of this vital on-going research, but vice president Jo-Anne Basile made it clear that the CTIA would not fund any post-market surveillance because cell phones were not pharmaceutical drugs.

In 2000, the industry was given another opportunity to prove safety when the FDA and the CTIA signed the Cooperative Research and Development Agreement (CRADA). Carlo outlines the inexplicable contract, "Under the government-industry research agreement there would be no new animal studies and none of the human studies that the government itself had once considered vital. And there would be no tracking and monitoring of the long-term health of people who use mobile phones." Under the provisions of CRADA, "the government agreed that the cell phone industry would pay for all the research studies - and what the industry would get for its money was the right to make all final decisions about which studies would be done and which scientists would do them. The industry and its designated scientists would also have the final say on whether and when the findings would be published." Carlo adds that, "In the executive branch and in congress, the watchdogs that

---

[78] Robert Kane, *Cellular Telephone Russian Roulette* (New York, NY: Vantage Press, 2001), p. 212.

70

were supposed to protect the public interest...never barked. They have failed to warn the people they are paid to serve."[79]

Lloyd's of London Rejects Industry

Did you know that Lloyd's of London, the world's largest risk takers, have declined to insure the cell phone industry against users' potential health claims? Due to a genuine concern of cell phone safety and the copious and serious health risks linked to cell phone use, John Fenn, a Lloyd's of London representative from the Stirling underwriting group, has refused to insure cell phone manufacturers against health-related claims. Numerous studies indicating a strong correlation between cell phone use and the development of tumors, cancer, brain damage, and Alzheimer's, are apparently too perilous for the company to accept. Lloyd's of London insured the tobacco industry and it seems they are unwilling to make the same mistake twice.[80]

Furthermore, even as the industry continues to convince you of cell phone safety, manufacturers are simultaneously and secretly administering a strategy that entirely contradicts it. In the early months of 2007, during a conference call with Dr. Carlo, it was disclosed that the cellular industry has set up a $6 billion dollar insurance fund of its own to pay for health related law suits, which are likely to arise in the future.[81]

That's odd. Why would a multi-billion dollar insurance account need to be established for something that, by all accounts, shouldn't be an issue?

---

[79] George Carlo and Martin Schram, *Cell Phones: Invisible Hazards of the Wireless Age* (New York, NY: Carroll & Graf Publishers, 2001), pp. XIII, 139-141.
[80] Ryle, Sarah, "UK Insurers Balk at Risks of Phones", *The Observer*, http://www.goaegis.com/articles/observer_041199.html
[81] Carlo, George, conference call via BIOPRO International, Inc. (January 2007).

CHAPTER 6

Hidden Health Hazards

What Americans are not being told, is that 3 out of 4 independent, scientific global research studies show adverse biological effects resulting from low-level, non-ionizing microwave radiation, like that which emanates from cell phones. Even conservative researchers believe that such effects are "probable", much more likely to occur than by mere possibility or random chance.[82]

Also hidden from consumers is the fact that for three decades between 1960 and 1990, over 40 studies confirmed and clearly demonstrated that RF/MW radiation does have an adverse biological health effect on human beings.[83]

Regardless of what you currently choose to believe or not believe, one thing is certain. Until objective investigative studies proving safety are conducted and confirmed, cell phone users are involuntarily participating as test subjects for what could be one of the world's largest research efforts of our time.[84]

---

[82] Glaser, Margaret Meade, "What Americans Need to Know about Radiation (or EMR) from Wireless Communications," *The EMR Network*, http://www.emrnetwork.org

[83] Cherry, Neil, *Neurological Effects of Radiofrequency Electromagnetic Radiation*, "Health Effects Associated with Mobile Base Stations in Communities: the Need for Health Studies," http://www.mapcruzin.com/news/cell062501d.htm (June 8, 2000).

[84] Philips, Alasdair, "Adverse Health Concerns of Mobile Phones", *Australia's Powerwatch Network*, http://frontpage.simnet.is/vgv/alist.htm

The Human Body

Over the past 60 years the world, which began with a natural static field of background radiation, has evolved into an oscillating field of electromagnetic radiation (EMR). The EMR and the wireless RF/MW radiation that the human body is now being exposed to originated when information was converted into waves being transmitted to and from close range antennas, or, in layman's terms, with the development of radio and television. Since then, the human body has been increasingly barraged with RF signals and microwaves from countless other sources.

Wireless technologies used to transmit and receive signals from cell phones, cell towers, Internet connections like Wi-Fi, satellite, radar, and other similar apparatuses, all significantly impact the environment, the body, and its state of well-being. The rapid advancement in the number of these manmade devices, accompanied by their radiating signals, has increased your exposure to 10,000 times more than that of your ancestors.

According to Dr. Neil Cherry, a leading New Zealand physicist in this particular area, oscillating fields emitted from wireless technologies are unnatural and unlike the normal static fields which are naturally present. While the human body is able to accommodate natural fields, oscillating fields interfere with the body's normal functioning and change cell behavior. Cherry explains how such abnormalities occur: "Biology reveals that brains, hearts and cells use electromagnetic signals, charged ions, voltage-gated ion channels, ion regulated gap junctions, all of which can be interfered with by external electromagnetic fields in subtle but vital ways in relation to health." [85]

Lest there be any unnecessary confusion, the EMR spectrum *includes* RF/MW radiation. Multiple studies have shown that cell phone radiation "mimics" EMR, both biologically and physiologically. Therefore, the previous statement could plausibly infer that external radiation fields, including those from cell phones,

---

[85] Cherry, Neil *"Evidence that Electromagnetic Radiation is Genotoxic: The Implications for the Epidemiology of Cancer and Cardiac, Neurological and Reproductive Effects,"* Extended from a paper presented to the conference on Possible Health Effects on Health of Radiofrequency Electromagnetic Fields, 29th June 2000, European Parliament, Brussels. *Cherry Environmental Health Consulting,* http://www.neilcherry.com

cell towers, and other external RF/MW radiation fields, interfere with critically necessary signaling channels in the human body.

This same electromagnetic interference is what causes the disruption or encumbrance of computers and other electronic equipment, in various situations. It is precisely why cell phone use is prohibited in hospitals and during aircraft take-off and landing. Cell phone communication signals can adversely affect the performance of electrically sensitive medical equipment, as well as cause static interference, disturb, or obstruct wireless communication signals to and from the air traffic control tower.

Compare these external examples of interference with the various ways the electronically sensitive human body can be internally affected by wireless signal exposure.

Identifying Problems

The biological effects experienced from RF/MW radiation exposure are dependent on a variety of factors. Frequency, duration, intensity, waveform, and power all play a key role in determining the effect that obtrusive exposure will have on various parts of the human body. It's quite possible that small amounts of this type of energy can have the same impact as massive doses, when delivered in the appropriate manner.[86] And contrary to the widely held assumption that older analog signals are more dangerous than newer digital signals, digital GSM phones emit pulsed microwaves which are biologically more interactive than the continuous wave of analog phones at the same frequency and power level. Digital phone pulses attack the user's brain cells at a rate of 217 times per second, and these pulses aren't exclusive to users. They also interfere with all who are in close proximity.[87]

Microwave radiation emissions have been found to promote stress, cause damage, and induce disease, as well as dysfunction. During the first 60-90 seconds of cell phone exposure three detrimental effects transpire. First, tissue and cell damage occurs, causing destruction and death of cells. Second, there is a repression of normal cell growth, and, third, an increase in membrane

---

[86] Begich, Nick and Roderick, James, *Earthpulse Press, Inc.*, "Cell Phone Convenience or 21st Century Plague?," http://www.earthpulse.com/products/cellphoneplague.htm (July 2004).
[87] Philips, Alasdair, "Adverse Health Concerns of Mobile Phones", *Australia's Powerwatch Network,* http://frontpage.simnet.is/vgv/alist.htm

penetration takes place. There is also evidence that the enzymes and proteins necessary for repairing damaged and abnormal cells, along with DNA strand breaks, become depressed and inoperable.[88]

In April 2001 the ECOLOG Institute in Hanover, Germany reported their findings on a study carried out by the German cell phone service provider T-Mobil. Physicists, medical scientists and biologists were enlisted to participate in the comprehensive study where numerous observations were made regarding the impact of cell phone RF/MW radiation on the human body. Their conclusions resembled those of other well respected researchers. "Experiments on cell cultures yielded clear evidence for genotoxic effects…like DNA breaks and damage to chromosomes, so that even a cancer-initiating effect cannot be excluded any longer." Cell transformation, cell promotion, and cell communication, as well as "disturbances of other cell processes, like the synthesis of proteins and the control of cell functions by enzymes, have been demonstrated."

The T-Mobil study also discovered recognizable "…modifications of the brain potentials and impairments of certain brain functions", which included blood brain barrier permeability along with an obvious deficit in learning capabilities and other cognitive operations. "Evidence for disturbances of the hormone and the immune system(s)" were detected as well. Cell phone radiation exposure was also shown to increase the production of stress hormones and cause stress reactions. A reduction of the hormone melatonin, the body's most powerful antioxidant which regulates the wake/sleep cycle, was similarly observed. [89]

Another European study examined 70,000 cell phone users and found that 20% associated their recurring headaches and fatigue to exposure. The data also revealed that 47% who were on their phone for an hour or more a day experienced at least one of the following symptoms: dizziness, concentration difficulties, memory loss, or a burning sensation near the ear where their phone was held.[90] Other similar research projects have reported that 70% of cell phone users experience one or more of the following common abnormalities while on their phone: warmth around the ear, facial

---

[88] Robert Kane, *Cellular Telephone Russian Roulette* (New York, NY: Vantage Press, 2001), pp. 12, 20.
[89] Health Effects of Microwave Radiation (Western View), *http://www.Goodhealthinfo.net/radiation/health_efx_western.htm*
[90] Raloff, J., "Researchers Probe Cell Phone Effects," *Science News*, February 12, 2000.

burning or tingling, fatigue, headache, dizziness, discomfort, concentration difficulties, and memory loss. These symptoms have all been identified as early warning signs of what could result in permanent, irreversible neurological damage.[91, 92]

Dr. Kejell Hansson Mild of the Swedish National Institute for Working Life, along with an international advisory group, discovered that the symptoms of headaches, dizziness, feelings of discomfort (pain, anxiety, irritability, or moodiness), and difficulties with concentration were experienced in direct correlation with cell phone use. In other words, symptoms elevated in occurrence as the number of calls escalated and as time on the phone increased. From over 15,000 randomly selected cell phone users, the prevalence of symptoms was significantly raised by as much as six times.[93]

These types of problems are being reported all over the world by casual cell phone users. Complaints to the Powerwatch Network of Australia revealed that headaches are usually first to develop. Headaches are often followed by concentration difficulties and short term memory loss, both of which have subtle beginnings that increase with exposure. Then fatigue or excessive tiredness transpire and are likely to be accompanied by a tingling sensation or heating of the skin, eye spasms or buzzing in the head.[94] Symptoms that begin as neurological can advance to promote autonomic vascular changes, which can affect blood pressure, induce sweating, or result in skin rashes. Cardiac symptoms, such as heart pains or ECG alterations, can also develop.[95]

Other documented non-thermal biological effects, resulting from external exposure to electromagnetic fields, include: cell membrane permeability; alterations of the signal transduction processes, resulting in abnormal cell behavior; changes in calcium ions; ornithine decarboxylase, protein kinase C and cAMP activities;

---

[91] Salford, Lief, G. et al. "Nerve Cell Damage in Mammalian Brain after Exposure to Microwaves from GSM Mobile Phones," *Environmental Health Perspectives*, Vol. 111: pp. 881-883, 2003.

[92] Sandstrom, Monica, et al., "Mobile Phone Use and Subjective Symptoms: Comparison of Symptoms Experienced by Users of Analogue and Digital Mobile Phones," *Occupational Medicine* Vol. 51, 2001, pp. 25-35.

[93] George Carlo and Martin Schram, *Cell Phones: Invisible Hazards of the Wireless Age* (New York, NY: Carroll & Graf Publishers, 2001), pp. 118-119.

[94] Philips, Alasdair, "Adverse Health Concerns of Mobile Phones", *Australia's Powerwatch Network*, http://frontpage.simnet.is/vgv/alist.htm

[95] Sadcikova, M., "Biologic Effects & Health Hazards of Microwave Radiation", international symposium sponsored by WHO (World Health Organization), Warsaw, 1973. Warsaw: *Polish Medical Publishers*, pp. 261-267, 1974.

alterations in DNA synthesis; enzyme activity; ion transport; cell proliferation; and transformations in the entire cell cycle.[96] Additionally, numerous studies support a very significant increase in a wide variety of cancers and tumors, DNA damage, chromosome abnormalities, as well as frightening consequences to the neurological, cardiovascular, reproductive, respiratory, digestive, hormonal, and immune systems.

It is important to recognize that a number of the above mentioned effects have been found to occur at levels far below those that are considered safe by the U.S. government. That is to say, that many of these detrimental consequences transpire at exposure levels 100 to 1000 times below FCC safety standards.[97]

Are You Sick?

Do you suffer from headaches? Migraines? Fatigue? Depression? Anxiety? Irritability? Dizziness? Nausea? Blood pressure alterations? Tinnitus? Impotence? Infertility? Insomnia? Concentration problems? Learning difficulties? Forgetfulness? Memory loss? or Confusion?

You are not alone. Globally, millions of people suffer and take medication for one or more of these identical symptoms. Although there are multiple sources which can elicit these types of bodily reactions, each and every one of these seemingly unrelated ailments has been shown to be a direct consequence of RF/MW radiation exposure. When you are sick, you go through a process of elimination to identify the root cause or irritant of your dilemma; what you discover and the decisions you make regarding that discovery can often put you on the road to recovery. Consider taking a closer look into this, because you may have a medical condition known as Microwave Sickness, which was introduced in the previous chapter.

The most common symptoms of Microwave Sickness are: chronic excitation of the sympathetic nervous system or stress

---

[96] Philips, Alasdair, "Adverse Health Concerns of Mobile Phones", *Australia's Powerwatch Network,* http://frontpage.simnet.is/vgv/alist.htm

[97] Cherry, Neil *"Evidence that Electromagnetic Radiation is Genotoxic: The Implications for the Epidemiology of Cancer and Cardiac, Neurological and Reproductive Effects,"* Extended from a paper presented to the conference on Possible Health Effects on Health of Radiofrequency Electromagnetic Fields, 29th June 2000, European Parliament, Brussels. p. 34. *Cherry Environmental Health Consulting,* http://www.neilcherry.com

syndrome; high blood pressure; headaches; dizziness; eye pain; sleeplessness; irritability; anxiety; stomach pain; nervous tension; concentration difficulties; hair loss; increased risk of cataracts; appendicitis; reproductive problems; extreme exhaustion; heart disease; heart attack; and cancer.[98]

Although the name and existence of this disease may be unfamiliar to you and your doctor, it's very likely that you or someone you know is struggling with any one or more of these symptoms as a result of RF/MW exposure. The development of Microwave Sickness is characterized by changes in brain activity and EEG patterns. These are typically followed by an attack on the central nervous system.[99]

Despite the fact that the vast majority of western physicians remain unaware of the existence of Microwave Sickness, medical experts in many other parts of the world are recognizing, diagnosing, and treating this monumental epidemic. However, if you question the validity of the illness, allow me to share a personal experience with you.

While Steve and I were searching for answers, his primary care physician sold his practice. You can't imagine how excited I was to learn that the doctor who bought the practice had studied in Russia. I was sure that he was the answer to our prayers after I called his office and learned that he was very familiar with Microwave Sickness. An appointment could not be scheduled soon enough.

When we were finally able to meet with the young professional, I asked him to educate us on all he knew about the disease. He gave us an ear full over the next 15 minutes, mainly because I asked question after question. He was happy and willing to discuss his expertise in this area and I thought: "Finally, we have a doctor who understands Steve's problem and will find us the help we need."

As soon as he finished talking, I dropped the bomb. "We need your help," I confessed.

The smile on his face and the enthusiasm with which he had shared his knowledge instantly faded. He looked at both Steve and me sternly. Then, as if to defend himself he put both of his hands up

---

[98] Hocking, B., "Microwave Sickness: A Reappraisal," *Occupational Medicine* Vol. 51: pp. 66-69, 2001.
[99] Cherry, Neil, *"Cell Phone Radiation Poses a Serious Biological and Health Risk,"* http://www.buergerwelle.de/pdf/cell_phone_radiation_poses_a_serious_biolo gical_and_health_risk.pdf (May 7, 2001).

in front of his chest as to push away the idea and a frightened look made its way to his face as he headed toward the door. He spoke firmly and very adamantly. "No, no. I can not help you. No, not here in the United States. No, no." We were dumbfounded as he quickly exited the room.

Needless to say, both of us we were extremely taken back, confused, and discouraged. I was appalled that, as a medical professional, he was not only familiar with the disease, but he had the answers we'd been searching for. Yet because of his geographic location, he was opposed to providing us with any assistance. For me, his unusual and seemingly fearful response clearly demonstrated how strongly RF/MW exposure and the known adverse health effects were connected, and how fiercely the information was being concealed from the American people.

As represented in the previous section, studies continue to validate the existence of the illness known as Microwave Sickness. Updated research offers a collective list of most all of the hidden health hazards which are known to result from RF/MW radiation exposure. They include, but are not limited to:

- Brain Activity Alterations
- Slowing of Reaction Time
- Memory Loss
- Anxiety
- Depression
- Irritability
- Hearing Abnormalities
- Vision Problems
- Motor Skill Loss
- Concentration and Learning Difficulties
- Nausea
- Sleep Disturbances
- Passivity
- Blood Pressure Alterations
- Behavioral Changes
- Convulsions

80

Presently, it is estimated that over 3% of Sweden's population, more than 285,000 people, have been diagnosed as electro sensitive, because of increased amounts of EMF (electromagnetic fields) in their environment. RF/MW radiation falls into the same electromagnetic category as EMF and EMR, it thereby duplicates its adverse biological effects so much so that Swedish victims experience symptoms identical to those of Microwave Sickness sufferers.

The Swedish Government has even gone so far as to recognize the illness as such a debilitating condition that those affected are entitled to compensation under a plan similar to that of the U.S. Social Security/Disability Program.

Similarly, over 2 million people in Britain suffer from these same symptoms and have been identified as being electro sensitive.[100]

Unfortunately, Americans who are electro sensitive or who have developed Microwave Sickness are destined to suffer alone in their misery. From a personal standpoint, I know just how devastating this can be for a person. It is unbelievably frustrating not only to function under such conditions, but to try and get others to understand your circumstances, so that proper care can be obtained. Both of these diseases are seriously debilitating, robbing people of the dignity and the quality of life they once treasured.

Damaging Effects are Rarely Immediate

The fact that RF/MW radiation is non-thermal and doesn't always generate initial adverse reactions, presents another form of deception, one that is self-imposed. Operators assume that if they don't suffer from any immediate symptoms, they're probably not being affected. However, the preliminary development of long-term damaging effects is often unnoticeable, because they seldom occur instantaneously. As with the development of any adverse health condition, individual results vary in terms of time, degree of exposure, and intensity.

Whether or not your body has an instantaneous reaction to your phone's emissions, Dr. Kane and other experts know that there is one thing you can be sure of. "If a cellular telephone operator picks up a portable and makes a call it should be with the knowledge

---

[100] Raising awareness of the harmful effects of cell phone masts: http:// www.Mast-Victims.org (2006).

81

that he will also be modifying the functioning of his brain for about the next week. Every action that occurs in that individual's life during that next week will be affected by the EEG modifications resulting from the portable cellular telephone call." EEG alterations in the brain are experienced as memory loss, mood swings, and a decrease in motor skill ability.[101]

It is critical to understand that, even though you may not experience any blatant exposure-related effects immediately, irreversible damage can begin to establish itself without your knowledge or awareness. Effects often start so subtly that once the problem is finally identified; there is little that can be done to correct it.

According to a 36 year compilation of Russian scientific studies (1960-1996) known as the Russian Medical Literature, it was discovered that both objective and subjective exposure symptoms are cumulative in nature. The data extracted from this thorough investigative anthology indicated that subjects experienced little to no effect within the first three years of exposure. However, the severity and frequency of symptoms increased with exposure; between the third and fifth year symptoms emerged and gradually increased. Following the fifth year of exposure ailments became more intense and continued to persist.

It was also reported that early exposure symptoms, those which occurred within the first five years, were reversible and could even be eliminated if exposure was reduced or avoided. Conversely, after five years of exposure, symptoms remained, increased in intensity, and became permanent. At this time, it was found that neither an exposure reduction nor complete avoidance could revert the victim to a previous state of well being.

Contrary to what the industry wants you to believe, scientists and researchers began studying the effects of non-ionizing radiation long before cell phones came into existence. As early as the late 1960s, numerous studies repeatedly revealed that even small doses of low level, cell phone type RF/MW radiation could cause adverse health effects.

---

[101] Robert Kane, *Cellular Telephone Russian Roulette* (New York, NY: Vantage Press, 2001), p. 100.

Substantiated evidence of the following consequences is undeniable. Cell phone RF/MW radiation exposure is known to:

- Heat the Head
- Penetrate the Blood-Brain Barrier
- Damage Brain Tissue
- Disrupt Brain Activity
- Alter Brain Waves
- Distort Brain Chemistry
- Damage DNA
- Reverse Cell Membrane Polarity

For the remainder of this chapter, along with the next three, the focus will be to identify the adverse health effects which have been shown to elicit a recognizable, significant, or dose-response impact on the human body as a result of EMF and RF/MW radiation exposure. According to over 1500 studies, which make up the Russian Medical Literature, the abnormalities which are likely to develop within the first 3-5 years are identified by an asterisk *. Those which are unmarked take longer to evolve.[102]

Physical Concerns:

Deterioration of Physical Capabilities*
The deterioration of physical capabilities can easily be attributed to neurological impairments, which are known to occur as a result of low intensity RF/MW radiation exposure. A decrease in motor skill ability, a slowing of reaction times, significant behavioral changes, and memory loss are some of the first physical signs to develop from exposure.

Hair Loss
Hair loss is a common response to cancer radiation treatments. It has also been shown to transpire as a result of RF/MW

---

[102] Maisch, Don, *"Biological Effects of Electromagnetic Fields on Humans in the Frequency Range 0 to 3 GHz: Summary and Results of a Study of Russian Medical Literature from 1960-1996,"* presented to the 10th International Montreux Congress on Stress, Montreux, Switzerland, Feb. 28-March 5, 1999. *Citizens' Initiative Omega*, www.grn.es/electropolucio/omega138.htm

radiation exposure. Although according to research, this consequence usually takes over five years to manifest.

Premature Aging

Some scientists believe that constant cell phone use causes premature aging. Dr. David Pomerai, head of the research team at Nottingham University's School of Biological Sciences, states that: "Low level radiation from the phone 'heats up' body cells, damages skin, and makes the user look lined and haggard." He goes on to say that: "Heavy mobile phone users are just like heavy smokers, who constantly inhale cell-damaging toxins without allowing the body time to repair the harm."[103]

Dr. Leif Salford, neurosurgeon at Lund University in Sweden, along with biophysicist, Dr. Bertil Persson and Dr. Neil Cherry all acknowledge that low doses of microwave radiation from GSM (digital) phones and other sources contribute to premature aging.[104] Evidence of increased cell death and cell damage, along with the reduction of melatonin which increases free radicals, both resulting from RF/MW radiation exposure, accelerates the aging process which promotes premature aging. [105, 106]

Thyroid Hyperfunction*

Thyroid Hyperfunction, also known as Hyperthyroidism, results from the overproduction of thyroid hormones. Thyroid hormones influence the body's metabolic processes. This abnormality can initiate a variety of disorders, including the development of Grave's disease, toxic adenomas, sub acute thyroiditis, pituitary gland malfunction, and cancerous growths in the thyroid gland.

---

[103] "Using a Cell Phone Makes You Age Faster," *Daily Mail*, October 18, 1999. http://www.earthpulse.com/src/subcategory.asp?catid=4&subcatid=3

[104] "Swedes Find GSM Radiation Causes Nerve Damage at Very Low Doses," *Microwave News*, Vol. 23, No. 1, January/February 2003.

[105] Cherry, Neil *"Evidence that Electromagnetic Radiation is Genotoxic: The Implications for the Epidemiology of Cancer and Cardiac, Neurological and Reproductive Effects,"* Extended from a paper presented to the conference on Possible Health Effects on Health of Radiofrequency Electromagnetic Fields, 29th June 2000, European Parliament, Brussels. p. 14. Cherry Environmental Health Consulting, http://www.neilcherry.com

[106] Reiter, R.J., et al., "Melatonin in the Context of the Free Radical Theory of Aging," Ann. *N.Y. Academy of Science,* Vol. 786: pp. 362-378, 1996.

Burning Sensations

Non-thermal radiation doesn't usually produce a detectible heating effect. However, multiple studies have revealed and confirmed that cell phone users experience feelings of warmth, discomfort, pain, tingling, and burning on the face or near the ear where the phone is held. Manufacturers and service providers want you to believe that heating must take place before any damage can occur, but research indicates otherwise. Evidence supports findings that damage can develop within the first 60-90 seconds of cell phone exposure. Once heat, pain or dull, achy sensations are experienced, deep tissue damage has already been imposed.[107]

Rashes

Rashes from exposure can emerge anywhere on the body. My late husband, Steve, had a large rash on his back and a smaller one on his forehead. They were always visible, but when he was in close proximity of a cell tower being exposed to its powerful waves, his rashes would almost instantaneously turn bright red. Away from the irritant, the color would eventually revert back to its previous state; the rashes never disappeared.

Optical Concerns:

Eye Damage / Visual Disturbances

As you have learned, eyes are extremely sensitive to microwaves and readily absorb their energy. Studies have shown that low power, pulsed RF/MW radiation at levels considered safe, damage the cells covering and protecting the eyes.[108] Blurred vision has been identified as a result of exposure, especially continual exposure.[109]

---

[107] Robert Kane, *Cellular Telephone Russian Roulette* (New York, NY: Vantage Press, 2001), pp. 22, 24-26, 52.

[108] Kues, H. A., Monahan, J. C., D'Anna, S. A., McLeod, D. S., Lutty, G. A. and Koslov, S., "Increased Sensitivity of the Non-Human Primate Eye to Microwave Radiation Following Ophthalmic Drug Pretreatment," *Bioelectromagnetics* Vol. 13: pp. 379-393, 1992.

[109] Barbaro, V., Bartolini, P., Donato, A., Millitello, C., Altamura, G., Ammirati, F. and Santini, M., "Do European GSM Mobile Cellular Phones Pose a Potential Risk to Pacemaker Patients?," *Pacing Clin. Electrophysiology*, Vol. 18: pp. 1218-1224, 1995.

Cataracts

Cataracts, or the induction of lens opacities, have been found to develop as a result of acute, high levels of RF exposure.[110] In 1959, Milton Zaret, a New York ophthalmologist, conducted a study for the Air Force to determine if there was a connection between radar exposure and eye problems experienced by military personnel. At first, there was no correlation between the two, but later it became apparent that the microwaves had deeply penetrated the eye tissue. Cataracts had developed behind the posterior capsule lens. Other research has concurred Zaret's findings. Airline pilots, air traffic controllers, and others who are heavily exposed are also at risk of developing this atypical eye condition.[111]

As a side note to optical concerns, it has been reported that cell phone users who wear metal-framed eyeglasses significantly increase their eye exposure, absorbing up to 60% more radiation than those who wear plastic frames or contact lenses. [112]

Auditory Concerns:

Hearing Disturbances & Tinnitus

Tinnitus, a hearing disturbance recognized as ringing in the ears, is a known occurrence that results from RF/MW radiation exposure. It has long been recognized beyond a reasonable doubt and seems to be widely accepted, since it is without much controversy.[113]

Dr. Allen Frey, a foremost authority in this area, was the first to discover and term the phrase "microwave hearing effect" in the 1960s. The microwave hearing effect produces both audible and inaudible noises that have been identified in a variety of ways - sounds ranging from ringing, to screeching, to buzzing, to hissing, to humming, clicking, or chirping.

---

[110] *ACN Online*, "Electrical Sensitivity: A Global Growing Concern. How Wireless Technology May Impact Child Development and Central Nervous System Functioning," Association for Comprehensive Neurotherapy.

[111] Becker, Robert, O., and Selden, Gary, O., *The Body Electric* (New York, NY: William Morrow and Company, Inc., 1985), pp. 307-308.

[112] Robert Kane, *Cellular Telephone Russian Roulette* (New York, NY: Vantage Press, 2001), p. 161.

[113] Petition for Inquiry of the EMR Network, Before the Federal Communications Commission, September 25, 2001, presented by attorney James R. Hobson, Miller & Van Eaton, P.L.L.C., Washington, D.C.

Strong signals can even produce sounds inside the head that are as loud as 120 decibels, which is equivalent to the thundering roar of a commercial jet taking off. Often, over-exposed people are subject to chronic, excruciating pain, caused by these irritating noises.

I can recall numerous episodes when Steve experienced the effects of microwave hearing. One night, while lying in bed, he commented on how loud the crickets were, but I didn't hear a thing. And there were several times when he'd walk into a room and ask if I had the TV or radio on. I never did, but he was always convinced otherwise. I also remember the days and nights when he would complain of high-pitched screeching that wouldn't quit. It was intolerable and kept him bed-ridden.

These agonizing and unbearable hearing disturbances are thought to be caused by rapid brain tissue expansion. Swelling occurs in the brain because of energy absorption and intense heating caused by radiation exposure. Microwave hearing effects occur at power density levels that are significantly lower than the current U.S. safety guidelines, levels that you are regularly and chronically exposed to.[114]

After years of studying various microwave frequencies, Frey determined that today's cell phones and their transmitting frequencies "fall in the most sensitive band for the microwave hearing effect." These same frequencies are also "in the band that has maximal penetration into the head."[115]

Perceptual Concerns:

Unprovoked Feelings

Frey also recognized that unprovoked feelings could be experienced by humans who were exposed to energy at frequencies within the cell phone range. Like sounds resulting from the microwave hearing effect, feelings can be perceived in a variety of ways, as well. Such impressions can be detected as minor annoyances (such as a tingling sensation similar to that of your foot falling asleep), severe, intolerable effects (such as a brutal buffeting

[114] Lin, J. C., "On Microwave-Induced Hearing Sensation," *IEEE Transactions on Microwave Theory and Techniques* Vol. 25, No. 7, July 1977, pp. 605-613.
[115] Frey, A. H., "Headaches From Cellular Telephones: Are They Real and What Are The Implications?," *Environmental Health Perspectives,* March 1998.

of the head), or anything in between the two extremes. Feelings experienced depend solely on the signal.[116] This reinforces the previously mentioned purposes for which international militaries are integrating this source of technology into the development of non-lethal weapons.

[116] Frey, A. H., "Human Auditory System Response to Modulated Electromagnetic Energy," *Journal of Applied Physiology* Vol. 17, 1962, pp. 689-692.

CHAPTER 7

Neurological Nemeses

Numerous worldwide research efforts have determined that RF/MW radiation elicited from cell phones induces significant changes in the central nervous system. The human brain operates using complex electromagnetic signals that transmit important information from cell to cell. These signals are electrically sensitive and are adversely impacted by even the smallest doses of external EMR.

From his comprehensive compilation of available research, Dr. Neil Cherry validated the fact that there is "a very strong and coherent set of data supporting a casual [extremely significant] relationship between ELF to RF/MW exposure, including cell phone usage, and neurological illness and death." [117]

Dr. Henry Lai summarized his observation in this way: "Existing data indicate that RFR (Radiofrequency Radiation) of relatively low intensity (SAR < 2 W/kg) [much lower than current standard safety guidelines] can affect the nervous system. Changes in blood-brain barrier, morphology, electrophysiology, neurotransmitter functions, cellular metabolism, and calcium efflux, and genetic effects have been reported in the brain of animals after exposure to RFR. These changes can lead to functional changes in the nervous

---

[117] Cherry, Neil *"Evidence that Electromagnetic Radiation is Genotoxic: The Implications for the Epidemiology of Cancer and Cardiac, Neurological and Reproductive Effects,"* Extended from a paper presented to the conference on Possible Health Effects on Health of Radiofrequency Electromagnetic Fields, 29th June 2000, European Parliament, Brussels. p. 49. Cherry Environmental Health Consulting, http://www.neilcherry.com

system. Behavioral changes in animals following exposure to RFR have also been reported."[118]

Since the central nervous system is one of the most sensitive systems in the human body, associated abnormalities are usually the first to develop as a result of exposure.

An asterisk * continues to be used to identify symptoms which are most likely to develop within the first 3-5 years of exposure, according to the Russian Medical Literature.[119]

*Delayed Reaction Time**

Slower reaction times have been identified in multiple studies as a direct consequence of the body's response to RF/MW radiation exposure. [120] Accompanying these findings is evidence that cell phone exposure delays the human "startle" response when surprised, alarmed, or taken off guard. In other words, acting quickly in situations which would normally provoke that type of response is inhibited.

This may not seem like a real concern, but consider what would happen in a dangerous situation. Suppose that, while you are driving, someone unexpectedly pulls out in front of you and cuts you off or a child runs into the road. Instead of immediately slamming on brakes, your response time is delayed. A few seconds could be the difference between life and death.[121]

This adverse effect alone could be one of the principle reasons why cell phone users have a higher than average accident rate. Research has shown that those who use cell phones while driving are 5.6 times more likely to get into an accident than those

---

[118] Lai, Henry, *"Neurological Effects of Radiofrequency Electromagnetic Radiation Relating to Wireless Communication Technology,"* Bioelectromagnetics Research Laboratory, Dept. of Engineering, University of Washington, Seattle, Washington. Paper presented at the IBU-UK Conference: Mobile Phones- Is there a Health Risk? Sept. 16-17, 1997 in Brussels, Belgium.

[119] Maisch, Don, "Biological Effects of Electromagnetic Fields on Humans in the Frequency Range 0 to 3 GHz: Summary and Results of a Study of Russian Medical Literature from 1960-1996," presented to the 10th International Montreux Congress on Stress, Montreux, Switzerland, Feb. 28-March 5, 1999. *Citizens' Initiative Omega,* http://www.grn.es/electropolucio/omega138.htm

[120] Cherry, Neil, *"Cell Phone Radiation Poses a Serious Biological and Health Risk,"* http://www.buergerwelle.de/pdf/cell_phone_radiation_poses_a_serious_biological_and_health_risk.pdf (May 7, 2001).

[121] Mitchell, C. L., *et al.*, "Some Behavioral Effects of Short-Term Exposure of Rats to 2.45 GHz Microwave radiation," *Bioelectromagnetics* Vol. 9, no. 3 (1988): pp. 259-268.

who don't talk and drive.[122] Accidents involving drivers who have an "active" cell phone in the car are also twice as likely to have a fatal outcome.[123]

*Slowing or Loss of Motor Skills**

Motor skills are activities that require the effective use of skeletal muscles to perform a particular task. Motor skills employ the use of the brain, skeletal muscles, joints, and nervous system. There are two types of motor skills, gross and fine.

Gross motor skills involve large muscle movements, using the arms and legs (i.e.: walking, stepping, lifting heavy objects, and physical exercise). Fine motor skills involve small hand manipulations, with an emphasis on hand-eye coordination (writing, coloring, picking up small objects, and cutting).

A slowing or loss of motor skills is characterized by instability and a lack of coordination. It has even been established that children living near radiating towers, where wireless signals are constantly exchanged, are slower in their reaction times and have less physical endurance than children who are not exposed to the same degree.[124] A consistent drop in performance levels has also been reported in highly exposed subjects.

*Memory Loss**

Memory loss, bouts of confusion, disorientation, and forgetfulness are all early warning signs of neurological damage and neurodegenerative diseases. Memory loss, both short and long term, has always been one of the most prominent symptoms of RF/MW radiation exposure and it is also found to transpire at radiation levels far below current FCC safety guidelines.[125] At a World Health Organization (WHO) sponsored symposium it was revealed that 55% of those exposed to microwave radiation experience memory loss.[126]

---

[122] Violanti, J.M. and Marshall, J.R., "Cellular Phones and Traffic Accidents: An Epidemiological Approach," *Accid Anal Prev* Vol. 28, No. 2, (1996): pp. 265-270.
[123] Violanti, J.M., "Cellular Phones and Fatal Traffic Accidents," *Accid Anal Prev* Vol. 30, No. 4, (1998): pp. 519-524.
[124] Kolodynski, A. A. and Kolodynska, V. V., "Motor and Psychological Functions of School Children Living in the Area of the Skrunda Radio Location Station in Latvia," *The Science of the Total Environment* Vol. 180 (1996): pp.87-93.
[125] Ibid.
[126] Sadcikova, M., "Biologic Effects & Health Hazards of Microwave Radiation", international symposium sponsored by WHO (World Health Organization), Warsaw, 1973. Warsaw: *Polish Medical Publishers*, , 1974, pp. 261-267.

Forgetting where you left your keys or who you were supposed to call can easily be dismissed with excuses of being stressed, too busy, or aging. When forgetfulness increases or the misplacement of objects begins to occur more frequently, it is a serious issue that should not to be taken lightly. If this condition is not addressed and exposure isn't reduced in a timely manner, memory loss can become a permanent dysfunction.

In 1994, Dr. Lai and his team were able to show that microwave irradiation had a significant impact on short-term memory. Rats that were previously able to run a maze with proficiency were no longer able to do so after being exposed to microwave radiation and their inability to recall well known territory persisted for five days, sometimes longer, even after exposure had ceased.[127] A later study, testing the effects of low-level microwave radiation on long-term memory, yielded results that validated and confirmed the previous research. Rats that were taught and had mastered a task were unable to recall what was previously learned. They were incapable of performing after being exposed to microwaves. Unexposed rats in the control groups of both studies were unaffected.[128]

Several other scientists conducting dissimilar studies arrived at the same conclusion; they proved that memory loss is unquestionably a product of RF/MW exposure.

It has also been observed that low intensities of RF radiation disrupt normal functioning of the hippocampus.[129] The hippocampus is located in the temporal lobe of the brain; it is made up of neurons and it controls learning and memory.[130] The hippocampus also determines which memories are retained and which ones are forgotten. Disruptions in this area of the brain could also be

[127] Lai, H., Horita A., and Guy A. W., "Microwave Irradiation Affects Radial-Arm Maze Performance in the Rat," *Bioelectromagnetics* Vol. 15, no. 2 (1994): pp. 95-104.

[128] Maisch, Don, "Mobile Phone Use: It's Time to Take Precautions," *Journal of the Australasian College of Nutritional and Environmental Medicine*, Vol. 20, No. 1, April 2001.

[129] Sage, C, "Reported Biological Effects from Radiofrequency Non-Ionizing Radiation," *Wave-Guide: Sage Associates Studies Matrix*, http://www.wave-guide.org.

[130] Hyland, G. J., "Physics and Biology of Mobile Telephone," *Lancet*, Vol. 25 (2000): pp. 1833-1836.

responsible for behavioral changes and learning difficulties, but most certainly memory loss.[131]

Another theory as to why RF/MW exposure promotes memory loss is that EEG alterations in the brain have been shown to take place at levels 10,000 times lower than what cell phone operators are exposed to. EEG modifications can persist up to one week after exposure and can easily account for memory loss.[132]

In 1999, Dr. Leif Salford, a researcher and neurosurgeon, along with his colleagues at Lund University in Sweden, found that problems with memory and its processing functions could result from the penetration of harmful substances into the blood stream through the blood brain barrier (BBB). Their research notes that diseases such as Alzheimer's and Multiple Sclerosis could have a direct link with the opening of the blood brain barrier, which occurs as a result of cell phone radiation exposure.

Increased forgetfulness and progressive memory loss characterize the early signs of these and other neurodegenerative diseases.[133]

Blood Brain Barrier (BBB) Permeability Increased

The BBB is an essential membrane made up of a thin layer of cells that surrounds the brain. It is a natural defense mechanism that acts as a filter, protecting the brain from harmful chemical and toxic invasions that can disrupt normal functioning and cause serious problems. While keeping danger out, the BBB allows necessary substances to pass through from the blood into the brain. The BBB is critical in regulating the central nervous system, so its breakdown is extremely significant and detrimental.

Cell phone microwave radiation has been proven to maximize penetration into the head and open up the BBB. This allows hazardous toxins, including the body's own albumin protein, to penetrate the brain. The unintentional opening and penetration of

---

[131] Tattersall, J. E., Scott, I. R., Wood, S. J., Nettell, J. J., Bevir, M. K., Wang, Z., Somasiri, N. P. and Chen, X., "Effects of Low Intensity Radiofrequency Electromagnetic Fields on Electrical Activity in Rat Hippocampal Slices," *Brain Res* Vol. 904 (2001): pp. 43-53.

[132] Von Klitzing, L., *"What May Be the Biological Relevance of Altered EEG-Signals in Man Induced by Pulsed EM-Fields?"* 16th Annual Bioelectromagnatics Society Meeting, June 12-17, 1994, abstract book, p. 70.

[133] Maisch, Don, "Mobile Phone Use: It's Time to Take Precautions," *Journal of the Australasian College of Nutritional and Environmental Medicine*, Vol. 20, No. 1, April 2001.

carcinogens through the BBB adversely affects the entire nervous system, provoking memory loss, headaches, and increased intracranial pressure.

Additionally, this consequence has been proven to increase the risk of developing neurodegenerative diseases, such as Alzheimer's, Multiple Sclerosis, and Parkinson's disease.[134] Further deterioration of this critical protective membrane can just as easily lead to brain damage, brain cancer and tumors.[135]

Dr. Leif Salford and his team saw the opening of the BBB after just 2 minutes of cell phone exposure.[136] This response occurred at exposure levels 4,000 times less than those considered safe by current FCC guidelines![137] Their research also reported that as exposure increased, so did the deterioration of this vital protective membrane.[138]

Headaches*

Headaches are one of the chief complaints of cell phone users. Often, they are the first symptoms to develop. Numerous reliable research studies have concluded that there is a very strong and undeniable correlation between the two. Almost 50 years ago, while researching microwave hearing effects, Dr. Allen Frey found that he, along with his human subjects, were experiencing headaches when exposed to microwave energy. Frey was the earliest pioneer to give scientific evidence to the headache phenomenon. He validated the fact that headaches are a direct result of, not just any microwave exposure, but "microwave energy exposure at approximately the same frequencies, modulations, and incident energies that present day cellular telephones emit." Since then, this observable fact has been repeatedly confirmed by a large number of worldwide studies.

---

[134] Harris, Sarah, "Now Mobiles Give You Kidney Damage," *Daily Mail,* Dec. 3, 1999.

[135] George Carlo and Martin Schram, *Cell Phones: Invisible Hazards of the Wireless Age* (New York, NY: Carroll & Graf Publishers, 2001), p. 109.

[136] Harris, Sarah, "Now Mobiles Give You Kidney Damage," *Daily Mail,* Dec. 3, 1999.

[137] Salford, L. G. , "Blood Brain Barrier Permeability in Rats Exposed to Electromagnetic Fields from a GSM Wireless Communication Transmitter," *Abstract in Proceedings of the Second World Congress for Electricity and Magnetism in Biology and Medicine,* Bologna, Italy, June 1997.

[138] George Carlo and Martin Schram, *Cell Phones: Invisible Hazards of the Wireless Age* (New York, NY: Carroll & Graf Publishers, 2001), p. 111.

Conclusive evidence proving that headaches are caused by cell phone use is substantiated in the reality that extremely small amounts of RF/MW radiation have been shown to open the BBB and affect the dopamine-opiate system in the brain. There is a large body of confirming data supporting the theory that both of these biological incidents, which can even result from brief exposure, can lead to headaches.[139]

Headaches, like other cell phone related abnormalities, have been shown to increase and intensify with use. Symptoms have been shown to compound by up to six times as usage increases from less than 2 minutes a day to 60 minutes a day. Similar results manifest when daily calls of less than 2 are compared to daily calls of 4 or more.[140]

While pain in the head is commonly referred to as a headache, what cell phone users may actually be experiencing is intracranial pressure which is a direct response to rapid brain tissue expansion. Swelling in the brain is an observable result of energy absorption and intense deep tissue heating elicited by RF/MW radiation exposure.[141]

Anxiety / Discomfort / Nervousness*

There is significant dose-response evidence from numerous studies validating abnormalities of discomfort, nervousness, and anxiety resulting from EMR exposure.[142] Anxiety, along with headaches, is another one of the first symptoms to be recognized as a result of cell phone radiation exposure. When unveiling the multitude of consequences, anxiety and headaches top the list.

Feelings of anxiety, discomfort, uneasiness, and nervous tension can stem from the fact that this unnatural, external stimulus

---

[139] Frey, A. H., "Headaches From Cellular Telephones: Are They Real and What Are The Impacts?," *Environmental Health Perspectives*, Vol. 106, No. 3 (March 1998): pp. 101-103.
[140] George Carlo and Martin Schram, *Cell Phones: Invisible Hazards of the Wireless Age* (New York, NY: Carroll & Graf Publishers, 2001), pp. 118-119.
[141] Lin, J. C., "On Microwave-Induced Hearing Sensation," *IEEE Transactions on Microwave Theory and Techniques* Vol. 25, No. 7, July 1977, pp. 605-613.
[142] Cherry, Neil "Evidence that Electromagnetic Radiation is Genotoxic: The Implications for the Epidemiology of Cancer and Cardiac, Neurological and Reproductive Effects," Extended from a paper presented to the conference on Possible Health Effects on Health of Radiofrequency Electromagnetic Fields, 29th June 2000, European Parliament, Brussels. p. 45. [Beale et al. (1997)].Cherry Environmental Health Consulting, http://www.neilcherry.com

not only increases stress, but it uncomfortably interacts and interferes with normal bodily processes and functions.

Stress

Being agitated or "stressed out" when the circumstances around you shouldn't be eliciting that type of response may not all be "in your head." Several studies have proven that cell phone radiation exposure induces stress. An increase in the molecular "stress response" has been observed in human cells immediately following cell phone exposure.[143] This is how cells respond to environmental attacks; attacks that are perceived as being damaging or life-threatening. This survival "stress response" should be yet another indication that RF/MW radiation exposure, which the body views as an adversary to fight, is harmful.

Dr. Peter French of the Centre for Immunology, St. Vincent's Hospital in Sydney, Australia, has led a number of experiments on both human and animal cell lines to uncover their response to mobile phone radiation. Through his efforts, he discovered that repeated mobile phone use induces the chronic production of stress proteins (heat shock proteins). This stress reaction elevates the risk of tumor and cancer development, speeds metastasis (the spread of cancer cells by way of the blood stream), and decreases the effectiveness of anti-cancer drugs.[144]

Exposure has also been shown to reduce the neurotransmitter, norepinephrine; low levels of norepinephrine increase stress.[145] Stress in and of itself can, and often does, attack the weakest part(s) of the body. In doing so, it can rouse an extensive array of health problems, both minor and major. Other correlating effects such as anxiety, irritability, and discomfort resulting from cell phone exposure can further aid in provoking a sense of stress (and vice versa).

---

[143] Lai, Henry, *"Biological Effects of Radiofrequency Radiation"*, Paper for the Scientific Workshop "EMF-Scientific and Legal Issues, Theory and Evidence of EMF Biological and Health Effects" in Catania, Sicily, Italy, September 13-14, 2002, organized by the Italian National Institute for Prevention and Work Safety. [De Pomerai et al. (2000, 2002)].

[144] Melbourne, Alan, *Problems with the Rationale of the Draft Standard,* http://www.ssec.org.au/emraa/rf/may.htm (May 11, 2001).

[145] Merritt, H., Hartzell, R. H., Frazer, J. W., *"The Effects of 1, 6 GHz of Radiation on Neurotransmitters in Discrete Areas of the Rat Brain,"* in C. C. Johnson and M. L. Shore ed., Biological Effects of Electromagnetic Waves, Symposium proceedings, L. Boulder, Oct, 1975.

Suicide

A number of studies have substantiated the fact that a dose-response relationship exists between increases in suicide risk and exposures to both ELF and RF/MW radiation. One such study set out to determine the risk factors of 8,190 participants - 2,842 were employees who had been occupationally exposed for between one and five years; 5,348 volunteers made up the unexposed control group. From these numbers, 536 deaths were the result of suicide, translating to a rate of over 18% in suicides of exposed workers.[146]

A similar study reported an even more worrisome suicide rate. RF exposed British radio workers and RF/MW exposed radar mechanics reflected a 53% increase in suicide; a 156% increase in suicide was found when compiling data on exposed telegraph radio operators.[147]

I can personally attest to the high level of suicide risk facing occupationally exposed workers; Steve was another statistic. When thoughts of suicide are accompanied with stress, anxiety, and depression, other recognizable symptoms of exposure, suicide risk is significantly greater.

While this research data provides strong evidence that chronic occupational exposure poses great risks to employees, what exactly constitutes "chronic exposure"? Who can accurately determine the number of minutes, the hours of talk time, or the amount of exposure to other wireless forms of communication it would take to heighten one's risk of suicide?

If the subject should ever arise, and I pray it doesn't, don't avoid confrontation. Suicide threats should be taken seriously. Discuss feelings and options. Get help. Don't delay.

Fatigue, Exhaustion*

Always being tired, never feeling well rested, or having a severe lack of energy constitutes fatigue and exhaustion. A combination of these two abnormalities is often medically termed CFS: Chronic Fatigue Syndrome. Characteristics that can accompany CFS include becoming increasingly passive or lethargic.

---

[146] Perry, F.S., Reichmanis, M., Marino, A. and Becker, R.O., "Environmental Power Frequency Magnetic Fields and Suicide," *Health Phys*, Vol. 41, No. 2 (1981): pp. 267-277.
[147] Baris, D. and Armstrong, B., "Suicide Among Electricity Utility Workers in England and Wales," *Br J Industrial Medicine*, Vol. 47 (1990): pp. 788-789.

Since the early discovery of Microwave Sickness, fatigue and exhaustion have been recognized as being an adverse health effect of RF/MW radiation exposure. Throughout the years these psychological symptoms have been confirmed and re-confirmed on tens of thousands of cell phone users. There is undeniable evidence proving that cell phone radiation causes fatigue and exhaustion. As with other symptoms, these ailments become evident and intensify with increased exposure.[148]

There are a number of factors that could contribute to this symptomology. First and foremost, when the body is under stress, whether induced by RF/MW radiation or not, it gets tired. Another contributing factor could easily stem from the fact that RF/MW radiation decreases the body's melatonin production. Melatonin is an essential hormone that, among other things, assists with the REM (rapid eye movement) sleep cycle. A reduction of melatonin not only causes the loss of essential deep sleep, but it also provokes other sleep disturbances, including insomnia. These undoubtedly result in unrest, fatigue, and eventually, complete exhaustion.

Here again, when abnormalities such as fatigue begin to develop, the majority of cell phone users tend to conjure up excuses as to the cause. They've been working too hard or there are too many things are going on. And, while these are plausible reasons for being overly tired, the truth of the matter is that they're probably not getting the body's required amount of deep sleep. Rarely is exposure from one's cell phone considered. Therefore, instead of reducing exposure, a doctor visit is scheduled and prescription drugs are administered. As you can tell by the aggressive media campaigns, sleep inducing medications are a hot commodity.

On the flip side, have you noticed the number of energy drinks and pills on the market today? Is it sheer coincidence that these energy boosters were never in such high demand before now, when exposure has all but depleted your get-up-and-go?

---

[148] Coghill, Roger, "Why I Believe That All These Items Should Carry a Health Warning," *Daily Mail*, July 17, 1998.

Depression

There is significant dose-response evidence that depression results from exposure to low levels of EMR.[149] Although there are different types of depression, all are characterized by intense sadness that lasts for long periods of time and interferes with normal, everyday life. If you or someone you know suffers from depression, you will most certainly agree that depression is truly a debilitating disease that not only affects the diagnosed individual, but everyone around them as well.

Anti-depressants, which are used to help people cope with depression, are very dangerous and the need for them has soared tremendously since the introduction of cell phones. The number of prescriptions given to American children alone was multiplied by ten times between 1987 and 1996. A more recent survey revealed a 50% rise in anti-depressant prescriptions given to children from 1998 to 2002. Even more concerning is that a drastic increase has taken place in children under six years of age.[150]

Concentration Difficulties* / ADD / ADHD

Concentration difficulties that are medically diagnosed as Attention Deficit Disorder (ADD) or Attention Deficit-Hyperactivity Disorder (ADHD) have never been as prevalent as they are today and prescriptions for these abnormalities are some of the most popular.

The ability to stay focused and to direct attention toward one thing at a time becomes increasingly challenged when we are exposed to low levels of RF non-ionizing microwave radiation. Several studies have concluded that cell phone and cell tower exposure significantly hinders one's capacity to fully concentrate on the task at hand.

Research has also found that children attending schools or living in close proximity to cell towers experience an elevated stage

---

[149] Cherry, Neil *"Evidence that Electromagnetic Radiation is Genotoxic: The Implications for the Epidemiology of Cancer and Cardiac, Neurological and Reproductive Effects,"* Extended from a paper presented to the conference on Possible Health Effects on Health of Radiofrequency Electromagnetic Fields, 29th June 2000, European Parliament, Brussels. p. 45. [Beale et al. (1997)]. *Cherry Environmental Health Consulting,* http://www.neilcherry.com

[150] Vedantam, Shankar, "Antidepressant Use in Children Soars Despite Efficacy Doubts", *The Washington Post,* April 18, 2004. p. A01.

of attention deficit.[151] It's distressing to realize that the younger generation is paying such a huge price for their involuntary exposure. Not only are they likely to suffer from concentration difficulties, but when accompanied with memory loss, this duo can easily lead to learning problems, stress, frustration, and a genuine, yet unnecessary, lack of success.

On October 9, 2002 twenty two German medical doctors from the Interdisciplinary Association for Environmental Medicine called for a ban on mobile phone use by small children and restrictions for teens, because the diseases they were seeing at an elevated rate had all been shown to be a direct consequence of wireless communication emissions. This group of medical professionals was collectively treating a greater number of young patients who were suffering from various neurological disorders, including those related to learning, concentration (ADD or ADHD), and behavior.[152]

Learning Disabilities

The basis upon which learning disabilities are founded is closely tied to memory loss, confusion, concentration difficulties, and behavioral problems, all of which are direct results of exposure to wireless signals.[153, 154] British military scientists, along with many other researchers, have discovered that low intensities of radio frequency radiation (RFR) disrupt normal functioning in the area of the brain that controls learning and memory.

Another reason learning disabilities are believed to exist is because exposure to microwave radiation reduces dopamine, norepinephrine, and serotonin. Dopamine is an essential neurotransmitter for learning and other cognitive abilities.[155]

---

[151] Sage, C, "Reported Biological Effects from Radiofrequency Non-Ionizing Radiation," *Wave-Guide: Sage Associates Studies Matrix,* http://www.wave-guide.org.

[152] Reported by the *EMR (Electromagnetic radiation) Network*: http://www.emrnetwork.org/news/IGUMED_enlish.pdf

[153] Tattersall, J. E., Scott, I. R., Wood, S. J., Nettell, J. J., Bevir, M. K., Wang, Z., Somasiri, N. P. and Chen, X., "Effects of Low Intensity Radiofrequency Electromagnetic Fields on Electrical Activity in Rat Hippocampal Slices," *Brain Research,* Vol. 904 (2001): pp. 43-53.

[154] Pryer, Nick, "Mobile Phones Can Affect Memory," *Associated Newspapers Ltd.,* July 16, 1998.

[155] Merritt, H., Hartzell, R. H., Frazer, J. W., *"The Effects of 1, 6 GHz of Radiation on Neurotransmitters in Discrete Areas of the Rat Brain,"* in C. C. Johnson and M.

Dizziness*

Since the discovery of Microwave Sickness, dizziness has also been recognized as one of the first symptoms to emerge as a consequence of RF/MW radiation exposure. Feelings of dizziness or vertigo remain a common complaint of cell phone users today.[156] However, as with other known symptoms, few are aware of the connection.

Sleep Impairments / Insomnia*

Sleep disturbances are frequently experienced by cell phone users along with those who live or work in close proximity to cell towers and their sites. Even low levels of EMR (electromagnetic radiation) have been shown to impact sleep patterns, sleep quality, and REM (rapid eye movement) sleep. REM sleep is essential for achieving a real sense of rest; it is the deepest form of sleep and relaxation.

You can be deprived of this essential mode of sleep for a short time, but extended periods of deprivation will cause you to be restless and irritable. You may even find that it is extremely difficult to function. Conversely, when you've had plenty of sleep, but still feel tired, it's undoubtedly due to poor sleep quality or a lack of necessary REM sleep.

Low levels of RF/MW radiation exposure causes notable reductions in melatonin and initiates the efflux of calcium ions. Melatonin is a naturally produced hormone that regulates our wake/sleep cycle and studies have concluded that there is a significant dose-response relationship between melatonin loss and sleep disturbance. However, when exposure ceases melatonin levels rise; this can help promote better sleep quality. [157]

Calcium ions are essential in transmitting nerve impulses, and after observing the abnormal behavior of calcium ions during exposure, top researcher, Dr. Ross Adey, expected the interference to

---

L. Shore ed., Biological Effects of Electromagnetic Waves, Symposium proceedings, L. Boulder, Oct, 1975.

[156] Harris, Sarah, "Now Mobiles Give You Kidney Damage," *Daily Mail,* Dec. 3, 1999.

[157] Cherry, Neil *"Evidence that Electromagnetic Radiation is Genotoxic: The Implications for the Epidemiology of Cancer and Cardiac, Neurological and Reproductive Effects,"* Extended from a paper presented to the conference on Possible Health Effects on Health of Radiofrequency Electromagnetic Fields, 29th June 2000, European Parliament, Brussels. pp. 47-48. *Cherry Environmental Health Consulting,* http://www.neilcherry.com

cause sleep pattern disruptions. The ill-suited combination of REM sleep loss, melatonin reduction, and the efflux of calcium ions results in the development of highly significant sleep impairments that could easily lead to insomnia, an abnormal inability to sleep.

Neurotransmitter Function Impairments

Neurotransmitters are biochemical substances which transmit or inhibit nerve impulses at a synapse. They are used to effectively communicate information between cells; synapses are the means by which such information is transferred.

Up to 60% of the synapses in the human body are regulated by gamma amino butyric acid (GABA). GABA is a brain chemical associated with the slowing or stopping of nerve activity and many neurological systems are regulated by GABA. According to a study conducted by Kolomytkin et al., GABA systems are very sensitive to RF/MW radiation and modifications of this brain chemical cause abnormal pathologies.[158] It has even been reported in WebMD Medical News that, "Impairment of the GABA system could overwhelm the brain with sensory information, leading to many of the behavioral traits associated with autism. Autism is characterized by communication problems, social impairment, and unusual or repetitive behaviors."[159]

Autism

Multiple epidemiological studies have revealed a dramatic increase in the incidence of Autism Spectrum disorders. According to the Center for Disease Control (CDC), in the U.S. 1 in 175 children has been diagnosed with autism. This rate has accelerated significantly from 1970 where only 1 out of 2,500 children suffered from the developmental disability. In 1999 that number rose to 1 in every 285. What began as a highly unusual disorder 38 years ago has soared to a universal malady which according to world reports,

---

[158] Cherry, Neil *"Evidence that Electromagnetic Radiation is Genotoxic: The Implications for the Epidemiology of Cancer and Cardiac, Neurological and Reproductive Effects,"* Extended from a paper presented to the conference on Possible Health Effects on Health of Radiofrequency Electromagnetic Fields, 29th June 2000, European Parliament, Brussels. p. 51. *Cherry Environmental Health Consulting,* http://www.neilcherry.com

[159] Boyles, Salynn, "Gene Interaction Linked to Autism Risk", *WebMD Medical News,* August 3, 2005.

suggests that autism accounts for as much as 45% of all new developmental disabilities.[160]

It is believed that RF/MW radiation exposure could have a substantial influence on this increased rise in autism. This could be due in part to the sensitivity of the brain chemical, GABA, along with the impairment of its system.

Brain Damage

Intelligence documents show that western governments have known that cell phone radiation causes brain damage for over 30 years, yet have hidden the facts proving it![161] Cell phone radiation seriously damages the neurons in the brain which can lead to permanent, irreversible brain damage. [162, 163]

Dr. Lief Salford, neurosurgeon and Dr. Bertil Persson, biophysicist, at Sweden's Lund University reported "highly significant evidence for neuronal damage in the cortex, the hippocampus and the basal ganglia in the brains of exposed rats". Brain damage became notably visible at a low SAR of 0.002 W/kg. "A clear dose-response relationship" was also revealed. In other words as exposure increased, so did the amount of detectable brain damage.

Likewise, Dr. Yngve Hamnerius and his team at Chalmers University of Technology in Goteborg, Sweden, observed brain damage in rabbits that had been exposed to pulsed GSM digital microwaves. Although immediate evidence was not realized, a delayed response was observed; three to four months later "morphological and biochemical changes became apparent".[164]

If early warning signs of neurological damage are ignored and exposure continues, injuries to the brain can compound and lead

---

[160] "Advice for Parents of Young Autistic Children," Autism Research Institute, Spring 2004. http://www.autism.com/autism/first/adviceforparents.htm

[161] Moran, Kathy, "Soviet Proof That Mobile Phones Do Cause Brain Damage," *Daily Express,* November 10, 1999.

[162] Salford, L., Brun, A., Eberhardt, J., *et al.,* "Nerve Cell Damage in Mammalian Brain After Exposure to Microwaves from GSM (digital) Mobile Phones," *Environmental Health Perspectives,* Vol. 111 (2003): pp. 881-883.

[163] Vandervorst, Andre, *"RF/Microwave Protection,"* TUTB Newsletter, June 2003 No. 21. p. 13

[164] Salford, L., Brun, A., Eberhardt, J., et al., "Nerve Cell Damage in Mammalian Brain After Exposure to Microwaves from GSM (digital) Mobile Phones," *Environmental Health Perspectives,* http://www. ehponline.org (January 2003).

to permanent, irreversible brain damage.[165] Brain damage can be characterized in a number of ways and any brain function can be disrupted by damage. Headaches, fatigue, concentration difficulties, impaired memory, faulty judgment, depression, irritability, emotional outbursts, disturbed sleep, diminished libido, difficulty switching between two tasks, and slowed thinking are all symptoms of brain damage.

Neurodegenerative Diseases

Alzheimer's, Multiple Sclerosis, Epilepsy, Lou Gehrig's and Parkinson's disease have all been marked as neurodegenerative diseases that are significantly impacted by RF/MW radiation exposure. There is strong and relatively consistent evidence proving that a relationship does in fact exist between exposure and these particular neurodegenerative diseases. Not only is the risk for developing any one of these life altering maladies increased by exposure, but once a condition establishes itself, its distinguishing characteristics increase at an unusually progressive rate.

Each and every one of these neurodegenerative diseases involves the death of specific neurons. Medical professionals and scientists who study Alzheimer's have documented proof that high levels of amyloid beta in the brain can lead to the development of this disease. ELF can increase the amount of amyloid beta in the brain. The risk of developing Alzheimer's is also significantly increased by the penetration of harmful substances entering the brain through the BBB, as well as the decrease in melatonin production. Melatonin plays a key role in delaying the onset of a variety of neurodegenerative diseases and minimizes their severity.[166]

Alzheimer's disease has escalated considerably over the past 20 years, so much so that it has gained recognition as being one of the top ten killers in the United States.[167] On June 12, 2007, USA Today featured a front page article revealing that while Alzheimer's disease has always been hereditary, targeting the elderly, younger people in their 40's, with no family history of the disease, are beginning to be diagnosed. "Of the 5 million Americans who have been diagnosed with Alzheimer's disease, it is estimated that over a

---

[165] Vandervorst, Andre, *"RF/Microwave Protection,"* TUTB Newsletter, June 2003 No. 21. p. 13.
[166] Sage, C., *The Bio Initiative Report,*
http://www.bioinitiative.org/report/docs/section_1.pdf (May 2008), p. 13.
[167] *Alzheimer's Association*, http://www.alz.org (2008).

half-million of them are under the age of 65." Researcher, Ron Brookmeyer of the John Hopkins Bloomberg School of Public Health in Baltimore, projects that 1 out of 85 people worldwide will fall victim to Alzheimer's disease in the next century![168]

Uncontrollable Shaking or Trembling*

Uncontrollable shaking and trembling is one of the most prominent symptoms of the previously mentioned neurological maladies, ALS or Lou Gehrig's disease and Parkinson's disease. Therefore, the fact that these symptoms are mentioned here should come as no surprise. Each symptom has been shown to be the direct result of various EMR exposures, including that from cell phones and cell towers. A definite dose-response relationship has also been found to exist. That is to say that increased exposure elevates risk.

Dopamine is an essential neurotransmitter in the brain that controls body movement, learning, and other important cognitive functions. There is evidence that dopamine levels decrease as a direct result of RF/MW radiation exposure and reduced levels of dopamine can produce uncontrollable muscle tremors and twitches.[169]

Seizure-like Activity / Epilepsy

Scientific research has revealed that epilepsy, characterized by seizure activity, convulsions, and periods of unconsciousness, is another neurological disorder that has been shown to have a dose-response relationship to EMR exposure. Some studies have even proposed that cell phone radiation exposure significantly increases the frequency of seizures in epileptic children.[170]

Dysesthesia

Dysesthesia is recognized as distorted or unpleasant sensations experienced by a person when their skin is touched. This has been identified in workers whose occupations exposed them to

---

[168] Fackelmann, Kathleen, "The young become the emerging face of Alzheimer's; those under 65 with the memory-robbing disease face stress of lost jobs and income," *USA Today,* June 12, 2007, A1 News.

[169] Raven, Johnson, Losos, Singer, *Biology, 7th Edition,* (New York, NY: McGraw Hill, 2005), p. 950.

[170] Thamir Al-Khlaiwi, *Omega News,* Association of Mibile Phone Radiation with Fatigue, Headache, Dizziness, Tension and Sleep Disturbance in Saudi Population, http://www.omega.twoday.net/stories/296447

radiofrequency radiation (RFR) and it is a common symptom of Microwave Sickness.[171]

Although this disorder is primarily a neurological abnormality, it will be revisited when sexual and reproductive consequences associated with RF/MW radiation exposure are discussed. Along with reduced libido and the threat of erectile dysfunction, dysesthesia inhibits the sexual experience.

---

[171] Hocking, Bruce, "Microwave Sickness: A Reappraisal", *Occupational Medicine,* Vol. 51 (2001): pp. 66-69.

CHAPTER 8

Other Serious System Disorders

Dr. Neil Cherry, physicist and highly respected elected official of New Zealand, has extensively studied how RF and electromagnetic radiation (EMR), including RF/MW radiation, impact the human body. Following years of investigative research, Cherry compiled thorough documentation of multiple studies specific to this topic.

On June 29th of 2000, he presented his findings to members of the European Parliament and attendees at a conference entitled, Possible Health Effects on Health of Radiofrequency Electromagnetic Fields. Cherry asserted that there are "many epidemiological studies showing dose-response relationships for cancer, cardiac, reproductive, and neurological effects." [172] In other words, these adverse health effects are subject to exposure and as exposure increases, the likelihood of incident simultaneously increases.

Cherry is not alone in analyzing the data; other experts in this field authenticate his educated conclusion. While it's recognized that exposures across the EMR spectrum, including RF/MW cell phone radiation, adversely affects the central nervous system, the cardiovascular system, and the reproductive system, evidence also demonstrates that this external energy also negatively interferes with

---

[172] Cherry, Neil *"Evidence that Electromagnetic Radiation is Genotoxic: The Implications for the Epidemiology of Cancer and Cardiac, Neurological and Reproductive Effects,"* Extended from a paper presented to the conference on Possible Health Effects on Health of Radiofrequency Electromagnetic Fields, 29th June 2000, European Parliament, Brussels. *Cherry Environmental Health Consulting,* http://www.neilcherry.com

the respiratory, digestive, urinary, and immune systems. Hormonal excretions are also impacted.

Cardiovascular Concerns:

Cell phone RF/MW radiation induces significant changes in the cardiovascular system.[173] Natural electric pulses that cause the heart to beat can be disrupted by a variety of electromagnetic signals. Microwaves from cell phones, wireless internet (Wi-Fi), and satellite transmissions can all impede the natural, rhythmic beat of the heart.

You may recall that melatonin is a vital hormone that is used to regulate the body's daily cycle of rest and activity. This powerful hormone also has multiple functions within the cardiovascular system. It aids in sustaining a rhythmic heart rate and, along with serotonin, regulates blood pressure. In addition, melatonin is responsible for signaling the calcium ions, which cause the heart to contract.

Exposure to all types of wireless energy decreases the production of these essential chemicals, and the results can be deadly. Inadequate amounts of melatonin and serotonin can cause the heart to slow down or speed up, thus increasing the risk of developing arrhythmia or heart disease. This disruption can also elevate blood pressure as well as trigger heart attacks.

Increases Blood Pressure

Blood pressure increases and heart rhythm alterations are proven to occur from exposures across the EMR spectrum. This abnormal functioning alone can unquestionably lead to the risk of heart attack, heart disease, and even death.

In 1998, German investigators, Braune et al., found that 35 minutes of RF exposure increased resting blood pressure.[174] Another study conducted in 1997 by Hermann and Hossman, recognized that the body's response to cell phone radiation not only increased blood

---

[173] Khudnitskii, S. S., Moshkarev, E. A. and Fomenko, T. V., "On The Evaluation of the Influence of Cellular Phones on their Users," *Med Tr Prom Ekol,* Vol. 9 (1999): pp. 20-24.
[174] "Mobile Phone Electromagnetic Fields Increase Resting Blood Pressure," *Lancet,* June 20, 1998.

pressure, but also resulted in the development of what could be considered high blood pressure.[175]

With these, and several studies providing convincing evidence that all RF, including that from cell phone exposure significantly elevates blood pressure, The British Stroke Association has given operators the following recommendation, "...we believe it would be sensible to minimize the risk".[176]

Altered Heart Rhythm & Rate

Dr. Ross Adey has documented evidence that cell phone radiation breaks down the binding of calcium to the surface of cells.[177] Calcium is essential for heart muscle contractions, these determine rhythm. In 1990, Schwartz et al. found that when frog hearts were exposed to RFR, at levels much less than those considered safe by U.S. standards, the movement of calcium was altered.[178] Wolke et al. discovered that calcium concentrations in the heart muscle cells of guinea pigs were also greatly affected when exposed to low levels of cell phone radiation. Calcium variations can alter heart rhythm and rate; they can also increase the risk of heart disease or induce heart attacks.[179]

Increased Risk of Heart Disease, Heart Attack & Heart Attack Mortality

In 1983 researchers Hamburger, Logue and Silverman saw a significant dose-response relationship between RF/MW radiation exposure and heart disease. Other studies, like that of Savitz et al., observed a highly significant dose-response relationship of mortality stemming from arrhythmia as it relates to heart disease and heart

---

[175] Hermann, D. M. and Hossmann, K. A., "Neurological Effects of Microwave Exposure Related to Mobile Communication," *J Neurological Science*, Vol. 152 (1997): pp. 1-14.

[176] *Microshield*, http://www.microshield.co.uk/research.html (October 2006).

[177] Keller, John, "Are They Safe?," *Wall Street Journal*, February, 11 1994.

[178] Schwartz, J. L., House, D. E. and Mealing, G. A., "Exposure of Frog Hearts to CW or Amplitude-Modulated VHF Fields: Selective Efflux of Calcium Ions at 16 Hz," *Bioelectromagnetics*, Vol. 11 (1990): pp. 349-358.

[179] Lai, Henry, *"Biological Effects of Radiofrequency Radiation"*, Paper for the Scientific Workshop "EMF-Scientific and Legal Issues, Theory and Evidence of EMF Biological and Health Effects" in Catania, Sicily, Italy, September 13-14, 2002, organized by the Italian National Institute for Prevention and Work Safety.

attack.[180] The epidemiological evidence is solid. From his extensive research, Dr. Cherry concluded that, "EMR across the spectrum increases incidence and mortality from arrhythmia related to heart disease and from heart attack." [181] That is to say, that exposure from wireless communication signals increases the incidence of heart beat irregularity and death resulting from it.

Additionally, it has been reported that exposure to cell phone radiation causes red blood cells to leak hemoglobin, the red matter of the red blood corpuscles. The build up of hemoglobin is also known to cause heart disease, which is also life-threatening. [182]

*Chest / Heart Pain**

Due to these abnormalities found to occur in the heart as a result of exposure across the EMR spectrum, chest and heart pain are very likely to be experienced by exposed individuals. This is not an uncommon symptom for anyone who suffers from irregular heart beats or arrhythmia, In fact, it's quite characteristic.

Pacemaker Interference

Since pacemakers operate so much like a real heart and RF/MW energy adversely interacts with the human heart, it would be relatively safe to assume that it might interfere just as easily with pacemakers. To establish relevancy, multiple studies have been performed over the years to determine what effect, if any, would take place in pacemakers exposed to cell phone radiation. Researchers have concluded that there is consistent evidence proving that radiant energy of this type does in fact interfere with pacemaker

---

[180] Savitz, D.A., Liao, D., Sastre, A., Klecjner, R.C. and Kavet, R, "Magnetic Field Exposure and Cardiovascular Disease Mortality Among Electric Utility Workers," *American Journal of Epidemiology*, Vol. 149, No. 2 (1999): pp. 135-142.
[181] Cherry, Neil *"Evidence that Electromagnetic Radiation is Genotoxic: The Implications for the Epidemiology of Cancer and Cardiac, Neurological and Reproductive Effects,"* Extended from a paper presented to the conference on Possible Health Effects on Health of Radiofrequency Electromagnetic Fields, 29th June 2000, European Parliament, Brussels. p. 52. *Cherry Environmental Health Consulting,* http://www.neilcherry.com
[182] Begich, Nick and Roderick, James, *Earthpulse Press, Inc.,* "Cell Phone Convenience or 21st Century Plague?,"
http://www.earthpulse.com/products/cellphoneplague.htm (July 2004).

performance. The interference experienced in most of the studies has not been slight, but significant. [183]

Research efforts have observed rhythm slowing, heart beat acceleration, and complete stopping. Obviously, these disturbances can lead to serious medical complications, including death. Due to the severity of these findings, pacemaker recipients are strongly advised to keep wireless phones as far away from their artificial heart as possible.

To close this section, please permit me to share another personal experience. While speaking with a female travel agent in Florida, I was asked if cell phone radiation could affect the heart. The woman was asking because she had been experiencing heart problems and chest pain for quite some time.

Before answering her question, I inquired further, asking if she wore the cell phone on her body, because that could make a difference. Her response took me quite off guard as she gingerly reached down into her shirt and pulled out her phone, "Yes," she retorted, "I wear it in my bra!"

I was taken completely off guard and astonished. In response to her question I answered, "Yes, there is proof that an active cell phone that close to the heart can cause heart or chest pain as well as other serious dysfunctions." Then I strongly advised her to keep that "thing" out of her bra and get a purse to carry it in.

Reproductive Concerns:

Consequences to the reproductive system have also been found to develop from RF/MW radiation emitted from wireless communication signals. Laboratory and epidemiological studies have demonstrated a wide variety of adverse reproductive effects, ranging from a decrease in libido and sex drive to those which are much more severe. Serious reproductive disorders linked to radiation exposure include impotence or erectile dysfunction (ED), a decrease in sperm count, a reduction in sperm quality, infertility, and an increased risk of both miscarriage and birth defects. [184] Three types of

---

[183] Cherry, Neil, *"Cell Phone Radiation Poses a Serious Biological and Health Risk,"* http://www.buergerwelle.de/pdf/cell_phone_radiation_poses_a_serious_biolo gical_and_health_risk.pdf (May 7, 2001).

[184] Cherry, Neil *"Evidence that Electromagnetic Radiation is Genotoxic: The Implications for the Epidemiology of Cancer and Cardiac, Neurological and*

cancer, which have shown to be elevated approaching significance in cell phone users, can also be considered under this heading: testicular cancer, cervical cancer, and breast cancer in both men and women.[185]

Sex Drive Reduction*

Studies have revealed that exposure to RF/MW radiation, at levels similar to those emitted by cell phones, reduce the male sex drive. Exposure induces behavioral and endocrine changes along with decreases in blood concentrations of testosterone and insulin. There appears to be a direct correlation between radiation exposure and male testosterone levels. Specifically, the greater the exposure, the more significant the decrease in testosterone released into the body's glands. Diminished amounts of testosterone reduce libido or the desire for sexual activity.[186]

In 2002, Santini et al. tested this theory to determine if similar problems existed in people residing near cell towers where chronic exposure was experienced. They discovered that those living within 300 meters (~328 yards) of mobile phone base stations frequently complained of fatigue and lacked a normal, healthy sexual urge, representative of a more significant decrease in libido than those residing farther away.[187]

Impotence / Erectile Dysfunction

Under the influence of EMF (electromagnetic fields), like those emitted from cell phones and site antennas, sexual function can also be impaired by changes in the nervous and neuroendocrine systems.[188] Since libido and testosterone levels have shown to be

---

Reproductive Effects," Extended from a paper presented to the conference on Possible Health Effects on Health of Radiofrequency Electromagnetic Fields, 29th June 2000, European Parliament, Brussels. p. 14. Cherry Environmental Health Consulting, http://www.neilcherry.com

[185] Cherry, Neil, "Cell Phone Radiation Poses a Serious Biological and Health Risk," http://www.buergerwelle.de/pdf/cell_phone_radiation_poses_a_serious_biological_and_health_risk.pdf (May 7, 2001).

[186] Navakatikian, M. A. and Tomashevskaya, L. A., "Phasic Behavioral and Endocrine Effects of Microwaves of Nonthermal Intensity." "Biological Effects of Electric and Magnetic Fields, Volume 1," (San Diego, CA: Academic Press, D. O. Carpenter (ed) 1994), pp. 333-342.

[187] Santini, R., Santini, P., Danze, J.M., Le Ruz, P. and Seigne, M., "Study of the Health of People Living in the Vicinity of Mobile Base Stations: Influence of Distance and Sex," Pathol Biol (Paris), Vol. 50 (2002): pp. 369-373.

[188] Matrix & Aires: Scientific and Production Association, New Medical Technologies Foundation. "Aires Matrix of Health Revolutionary Universal

significantly reduced due to exposure, problems such as impotence, also referred to as erectile dysfunction (ED), are likely to arise.

This problem may have existed for some men in the past, but over the last 20 years these sexual disorders have become increasingly prevalent in our society. Millions of men, and indirectly women, suffer from this dilemma. The demand for pharmaceutical drugs such as Viagra and Cialis has soared and continues to increase. It's difficult to believe that this widespread disorder, along with the growing need for aid, is sheer coincidence.

Decreased Sperm Count

Numerous international studies conducted over the past 20 years have demonstrated a continual decline in adult male sperm count. These changes are not perceived as being genetic; they are presumed to stem from environmental or lifestyle factors. It is thought that if this down turn persists at its present rate, within a relatively short period of time widespread male infertility may be witnessed.[189]

Fertility specialists at the University of Szeged in Hungary discovered a sperm count reduction of up to 30% in men who carry a cell phone on their belt or in their front pants pocket. Sperm count decreased in direct proportion to the amount of time the cell phone was next to the body, emitting its harmful rays.[190]

Fertility Reduction & Irreversible Infertility

If exposure decreases sperm count, the ability to conceive children is also reduced. In 1997 Magras and Xenos confirmed that even low doses of residential exposures, levels which are considered safe, produced observable adverse reproductive effects in mice. Those that were exposed became less productive over time and by the 5th generation the exposed mice had become completely infertile,

Approach to Treatment and Prevention of Diseases to Replace Out-of-Date Technologies," http://www.matrix.com.ru

[189] Shiva Dindyal: The sperm count has been decreasing steadily for many years in Western industrialised countries: Is there an endocrine basis for this decrease?. *The Internet Journal of Urology.* Volume 2 Number 1 (2004)..

[190] Fejes, Imre, et al., *"Relationship Between Regular Cell Phone Use and Human Semen Quality,"* paper presented at the 20th Annual Meeting of the European Society of Human Reproduction and Embryology, Berlin, June 29, 2004.

no longer able to produce offspring. This study clearly demonstrates a cumulative effect.[191]

Decreased Sperm Quality

While low intensities of non-ionizing RF/MW radiation have been recognized in the scientific community as adversely influencing sex drive, sperm count, and fertility, it has also been shown to decrease sperm quality. Sperm that is mediocre or inadequate in some way can jeopardize the success of creating a healthy embryo and delivering a normal, unaffected child.

In October 2006, Dr. Ashok Agarwal, Director of the Center for Reproductive Medicine at the Cleveland Clinic in Cleveland, Ohio, found a direct correlation between cell phone use and deviations in sperm quality. The data revealed evidence of highly significant sperm damage in men who exceeded 4 hours a day of cell phone use when compared to men who were on their phones less frequently.[192]

Another study conducted in 2008 by Agarwal, confirmed his previous findings. However this time, exposure levels seemed to be more relevant; instead of measuring exposure from cell phone usage near the brain where the phone is held while conversing, exposure mimicked that which would be absorbed into a man's testes when an active cell phone is carried in his front pant's pocket. This endeavor of testing close range exposure not only exhibited a decrease in sperm quality, motility, and viability, Agarwal also reported that the sperm of *all* participants displayed an average increase of 85% in free radicals. Free radicals have been linked to a reduction of sperm quality, as well as a variety of other human diseases, including cancer.

Agarwal believes that these observable findings may be the result of deep tissue heating, which is known to transpire from cell phone radiation, in the gonads. Increased temperatures can adversely

---

[191] Lai, Henry, *"Biological Effects of Radiofrequency Radiation"*, Paper for the Scientific Workshop "EMF-Scientific and Legal Issues, Theory and Evidence of EMF Biological and Health Effects" in Catania, Sicily, Italy, September 13-14, 2002, organized by the Italian National Institute for Prevention and Work Safety.

[192] Wayne Rash, "Cell Phone Use Affects Fertility, Study Shows," *EWeek.com,* Oct. 27, 2006.

114

affect sperm cells. Testes have also been recognized as absorbing radiation more readily than other parts of the body, elevating risk. [193]

Increased Miscarriage Risk

A heightened miscarriage risk has been proven to result from microwave exposure. In a study of 6,684 physiotherapists, who had performed 3 minute diathermy treatments on patients using non-ionizing microwave radiation, a highly significant dose-response relationship was observed. The women who had been exposed to the microwaves had an astonishing 28% increase of miscarriage in their first trimester.[194]

Increased Risk of Birth Defects
& Reproductive Abnormalities

DNA damage and chromosomal alterations have been shown to occur at various levels of radiofrequency exposure, including those specific to cell phones. Evidence reveals that RF/MW radiation exposure not only increases the risk of reproductive abnormalities, but it also inflates the threat of birth defects in unborn children.

U.S. scientists exposed more than 10,000 chicken embryos to cell phone radiation with seriously disturbing results. Following exposure, multiple birth defects were observed and a significant mortality rate was evident. British mobile phone specialist, Roger Coghill, said the findings are "enormously worrying."[195]

In 1991, Somosy et al. found that mouse embryos were adversely affected in much the same way. The radiation caused molecular and structural changes in their cells.[196]

Due to the deep concern of these, and other similar studies, some researchers are urging pregnant women not to use mobile phones until the risks can properly be assessed. The French

---

[193] "Cell Phones Can Affect Sperm Quality, Researcher Says," *CNN News*, September 18, 2008.

[194] Ouellet-Hellstrom, R. and Stewart, W.F., "Miscarriages Among Female Physical Therapists Who Report Using Radio and Microwave Frequency Electromagnetic Radiation," *American Journal of Epidemiology*, Vol. 138, No. 10 (1993): pp. 775-786.

[195] Coghill, Roger, "FED: Pregnant Women Warned to be Wray of Using Mobile Phones," *AAP General News*, May 1, 1999.

[196] Lai, Henry, *"Biological Effects of Radiofrequency Radiation"*, Paper for the Scientific Workshop "EMF-Scientific and Legal Issues, Theory and Evidence of EMF Biological and Health Effects" in Catania, Sicily, Italy, September 13-14, 2002, organized by the Italian National Institute for Prevention and Work Safety.

government has even strongly advised pregnant women to distance their cell phones from their bellies. [197]

Respiratory Concerns:

Breathing Difficulties

RF energy also has a profound impact on breathing. Captain Paul Tyler was director of the U.S. Navy Electromagnetic Radiation Project between 1970 and 1977. In his contribution to the book, *Low Intensity Conflict and Modern Technology*, he warned that, "It has been shown that normal breathing takes place at certain frequencies and amplitudes and not at others. Animals (like humans) forced to breathe at certain unnatural frequencies develop severe respiratory distress." Frequency irregularities can produce feelings of uneasiness and anxiety, which can lead to suffocation, even resulting in death.[198]

Digestive / Gastrointestinal Concerns:

There are a few digestive disturbances which have been reported to arise as a result of RF/MW radiation exposure. They include:

Peptic Ulcers[199]

Nausea
Loss of Appetite
Vomiting
Diarrhea
Irritable Bowel Syndrome

---

[197] "Eye on Europe," *Microwave News*, Vol. 22, No. 2 (March/April 2002) p.5.
[198] "Have the Radiofrequency Weapons Been Put to Use Yet?", http://www.wealth4freedom.com/truth/12/mindcontrol.htm (November 2002).
[199] Maisch, Don, *"Submissions to Standards Australia on Adopting the ICNIRP Radio Frequency Exposure Limits for Australia and New Zealand"*. "ICNIRP RF/MW Guidelines for Australia / New Zealand" Discussion paper (A), July 24, 1998.

Urinary Concerns:

Kidney Stone & Kidney Damage Development
The kidney and liver are more vulnerable to cell phone microwaves than other vital organs in the body, aside from the brain. All three readily absorb RF/MW radiation, thereby leading to the possibility of complications, problems, and even organ damage. As mentioned under Cardiac Concerns, the leaking and build up of hemoglobin is a reactive response to wireless energy. Not only is this adverse reaction known to cause heart disease, it is also recognized as promoting the development of kidney stones.

One of the primary reasons it is best to avoid wearing an "active" cell phone on your belt or in your pants pocket is because of its close proximity to both the kidney and the liver. The testes are also especially susceptible in this area of the body. [200]

Hormonal Concerns:

Hormones that regulate and perform specific, necessary bodily tasks become impaired when exposed to low levels of radiation across the EMR spectrum. Detrimental exposures have been shown to stem from a wide variety of sources, including emissions from high voltage wires, radio and TV antennas, cell phones and cell towers, Wi-Fi, satellite, and radar signals. Regardless of the source, there is little difference in the body's response.

Hormonal excretions that have repeatedly been shown to adversely be affected by such exposure include those of melatonin, testosterone, insulin, thyrotropin, and cortisol. The obstruction or fluctuation of any one or more of these five essential hormones, can lead to a multitude of health problems. However, the reduction of melatonin is the most important, because it can threaten your life.

---

[200] Begich, Nick and Roderick, James, *Earthpulse Press, Inc.*, "Cell Phone Convenience or 21st Century Plague?,"
http://www.earthpulse.com/products/cellphoneplague.htm (July 2004).

Melatonin Reduction

In the book, *Your Body's Natural Wonder Drug,* Professor Russell Reiter, Ph.D., one of the world's leading medical researchers on melatonin, identifies the various functions of this hormone as: regulating the body's wake/sleep cycle, assisting with healthy sleep, maintaining normal body temperature, reducing cholesterol, and lowering blood pressure. Melatonin is also responsible for triggering several secondary functions, including sending calcium ions to flood the heart causing it to contract and helping it to maintain regular, rhythmic beats. Melatonin strengthens the immune system and is the body's most powerful antioxidant, protecting cells from cancer-causing agents like free radicals. In addition, melatonin is recognized as a mood stabilizer, and has even been considered an anti-stress hormone.

With so many vital and life-sustaining tasks, it becomes apparent that a decrease in the body's production of melatonin, as a result of EMR and wireless exposure, significantly compromises health and the human physical condition.

Testosterone Reduction

As previously referenced under Reproductive Concerns, studies reveal that cell phone radiation reduces the excretion of the hormone testosterone, which regulates the sexual function in men. Low levels of this essential hormone significantly diminish libido and can cause impotence or erectile dysfunction.

Insulin Reduction

Insulin is a hormone which controls blood glucose levels and has extensive effects on metabolism and other body functions. The production of insulin has also been shown to be reduced as a result of RF/MW exposure. One study found a significant insulin decrease of 26% when exposed to levels considered safe by the FCC. [201]

Diabetes is a real health concern when the body produces less insulin than what is needed for proper growth and energy.

---

[201] Sage, C, "Reported Biological Effects from Radiofrequency Non-Ionizing Radiation," *Wave-Guide: Sage Associates Studies Matrix,* http://www.wave-guide.org.

Diabetes is a chronic condition that has impacted the lives 23.6 million Americans. It is the sixth leading cause of death in the U.S.[202]

Thyrotropin Reduction

Thyrotropin, a thyroid-stimulating hormone, regulates several metabolic and behavioral parameters. It controls such activities as food consumption, physical movement, and has qualities which act as a natural antidepressant. The reduction of this essential hormone can promote eating disorders, encourage fatigue, and can even evoke depression. Nausea, fatigue, and depression are all common subjective complaints of individuals exposed to both chronic and acute levels of RF/MW radiation.[203]

Cortisol Increase

Human subjects demonstrated a transient increase in blood cortisol when exposed to cell phone radiation.[204] Cortisol is a hormone that is released into the bloodstream whenever the body perceives and reacts to stress. It is responsible for stimulating the conversion of proteins to carbohydrates, raising blood sugar, and promoting glycogen storage in the liver.[205] Chronic elevations of this stress hormone influence mood and can induce depression, it also weakens the immune system.[206]

Immune System Concerns:

Biological effects from EMF exposure, like that of cell phones and their antennas, have been shown to interfere with normal

---

[202] *American Diabetes Association*, American Diabetes Association Health Reform Priorities, http://www.diabetes.org/advocacy-and-legalresources/HRP-executive-summary.jsp

[203] Gary, K. et al. J. *Pharmacol. Exp. Ther.* 305, 410 (2003); Sattin, A. J. *ECT.* Vol. 15, (1999): pp. 76 Steward, C. et al. *Neuroreport*, Vol. 14, (2003): pp. 687.

[204] Lai, Henry, *"Biological Effects of Radiofrequency Radiation"*, Paper for the Scientific Workshop "EMF-Scientific and Legal Issues, Theory and Evidence of EMF Biological and Health Effects" in Catania, Sicily, Italy, September 13-14, 2002, organized by the Italian National Institute for Prevention and Work Safety.

[205] *Biology Online*, http://www.biology-online.org

[206] Het, Serkan, MSc, and Wolf, Oliver T. PhD, University of Bielefeld, "Mood Changes in Response to Psychosocial Stress in Healthy Young Women: Effects of Pretreatment with Cortisol," *Behavioral Neuroscience*, Vol. 121, No. 1.

immune system functioning.[207] The overall impact these external stimuli have on the human body is subtle, yet devastating. The internal transformations that occur from exposure not only affect cells and tissue in a variety of ways, but they also play a key role in your ability to fight off and repair damage. Like so many other related symptoms, this occurrence takes place at levels well below those that the U.S. Government accepts as being safe. [208]

The critical malfunctions that threaten the immune system and one's overall well being can be primarily attributed to the fact that exposure has been proven to alter calcium ions and significantly reduce melatonin. Both of these abnormalities not only contribute to the development of a weakened immune system, but they also have other serious implications that create an adverse domino effect of threatening consequences.[209]

Additionally, there is substantiated evidence that, since the immune system senses danger and reacts accordingly to RF exposure, inflammatory and allergic reactions can also result. Chronic excitation of this nature can lead to immune dysfunction, chronic allergic responses, inflammatory disease, and ill health. [210]

Hodgkin's disease

Hodgkin's disease, sometimes referred to as Hodgkin's Lymphoma, is a cancer of the lymphatic system, which is part of the immune system. A number of heavy cell phone users who admitted to being on their phones for a minimum of two hours a day, developed Hodgkin's disease in their neck lymph glands. The disease appeared on the same side that users reported holding their

---

[207] *Matrix & Aires:* Scientific and Production Association, New Medical Technologies Foundation. "Aires Matrix of Health Revolutionary Universal Approach to Treatment and Prevention of Diseases to Replace Out-of-Date Technologies," http://www.matrix.com.ru

[208] Lai, Henry, *"Biological Effects of Radiofrequency Radiation"*, Paper for the Scientific Workshop "EMF-Scientific and Legal Issues, Theory and Evidence of EMF Biological and Health Effects" in Catania, Sicily, Italy, September 13-14, 2002, organized by the Italian National Institute for Prevention and Work Safety.

[209] Cherry, Neil "Evidence that Electromagnetic Radiation is Genotoxic: The Implications for the Epidemiology of Cancer and Cardiac, Neurological and Reproductive Effects," Extended from a paper presented to the conference on Possible Health Effects on Health of Radiofrequency Electromagnetic Fields, 29th June 2000, European Parliament, Brussels. p. 56.

[210] Sage, C., *The Bio Initiative Report,*
http://www.bioinitiative.org/report/docs/section_1.pdf (May 2008), p. 18.

phones while talking.[211] As Hodgkin's disease progresses, it compromises the body's ability to fight infection.

---

[211] Philips, Alasdair, "Adverse Health Concerns of Mobile Phones", *Australia's Powerwatch Network,* http://frontpage.simnet.is/vgv/alist.htm

CHAPTER 9

Genotoxic Damage & Cancer

Ever since 1993, when the cell phone industry was hit with its first cancer lawsuit, consumers have questioned whether or not cell phone use causes cancer. While it should come as no surprise that industry-funded studies continue to present inconclusive evidence of genotoxic damage and cancer risk, substantiated evidence of these adverse health effects continue to emerge from independent endeavors, generating an affirmative response to this lingering concern.

A long term research effort, which went by the name REFLEX (Risk evaluation of potential environmental hazards from low-energy electromagnetic field EMF exposure using sensitive in-vitro methods), was initiated to evaluate the risks and potential health hazards of environmental RF and EMF exposure, specifically from cell phones and their masts. Twelve scientists from seven European universities and organizations participated in the study, which ran from February 2000 through May 2004. The published findings revealed numerous atypical changes in biological functioning.

The abnormalities which relate to genotoxic damage and cancer formation found to exist in the REFLEX study are as follows:

> ➤ "Gene mutations, cell proliferation, and apoptosis are caused by or result in altered gene and protein expression profiles. The convergence of these events is required for the development of all chronic diseases."

> "Genotoxic effects and a modified expression of numerous genes and proteins after EMF exposure could be demonstrated with great certainty."

> "RF-EMF produced genotoxic effects in fibroblasts, HL-60 cells, granulosa cells of rats, and neural progenitor cells derived from mouse embryonic stem cells."

> "Cells responded to RF exposure between SAR levels of 0.3 and 2 W/Kg with a significant increase in single and double-strand DNA breaks and in micronuclei frequency."

> "In HL-60 cells an increase in intracellular generation of free radicals accompanying RF-EMF exposure could clearly be demonstrated."

> "The induced DNA damage was not based on thermal effects and arouses consideration about the environmental safety limits for ELF-EMF exposure." [212]

Dr. Graham Blackwell gave an account of this study in his article entitled The REFLEX Report. His statement read: "Based on the methodology used and the data obtained in the REFLEX study, the findings on genotoxicity caused by RF-EMF are hard facts."

Chromosome / DNA Damage

Numerous studies have revealed that chromosomes, the building blocks for DNA, are damaged when exposed to RF/MW radiation. Damaged chromosomes change the hereditary messaging of an organism. DNA damage alters the genetic code for growth and development. It also changes cells and diminishes their ability to perform basic functions. DNA damage transpires in a variety of ways; some even occurs naturally.

If new damage takes place before preexisting damage has been given adequate time to repair, injuries compound and negative consequences become elevated and increasingly obvious. Adverse effects which can occur as a result of DNA damage is deterioration of the organ(s) being attacked, the development of cancer, mutations,

---

[212] Sage, C., *The Bio Initiative Report,*
http://www.bioinitiative.org/report/docs/section_1.pdf (May 2008), pp. 16-17.

birth defects, immune system impairments, and other serious health complications.[213]

To make matters worse, not only has it been confirmed that cell phone radiation causes DNA damage, it has also been recognized that this same exposure reduces the cells' ability to repair any preexisting affliction.[214]

While these health conditions and malformations may not have a significant affect on you, if not adequately repaired, they, along with their associated abnormalities, will be passed down through the generations. Irregular genetic coding will be transferred first to your children. Then your children's damaged DNA will compound with yours and be passed on to your grandchildren. From there the domino effect continues.

This snowball of consequences isn't likely to change in the near future if this vicious cycle of increased technological exposure continues. Each generation will be faced with increased difficulty, fighting the odds of being born healthy and free of complications.

At this point it may be helpful to understand the domino effect that the reduction of melatonin has on chromosome and DNA damage. Cell phone radiation significantly reduces melatonin and the reduction simultaneously decreases the amount of antioxidants that are released into the body, causing free radicals to multiply. Instead of having ample amounts of melatonin to adequately protect the body from these harmful agents, free radicals have no restraints and actively seek to damage cells and destroy DNA.

Knowing that this type of damage occurs, whether related to reduced levels of melatonin or not, proves that cell phone radiation exposure is not only genotoxic, but carcinogenic, as well.

Gene Transcription Activity Altered

A number of scientific experiments have provided evidence that RF/MW radiation at cell phone frequencies significantly enhances and alters proto-oncogene activity.[215] Proto-oncogenes are normal genes that promote cell division.

---

[213] George Carlo and Martin Schram, *Cell Phones: Invisible Hazards of the Wireless Age* (New York, NY: Carroll & Graf Publishers, 2001), pp. 20, 63.

[214] Maisch, Don, "Mobile Phone Use: it's time to take precautions," *Journal of the Australasian College of Nutritional and Environmental Medicine*, Vol. 20, No. 1, April 2001.

[215] Goswami, P. C., Albee, L. D., Parsian, A. J., Baty, J. D., Moros, E. g. Pickard, W. F., Roti, J. L. and Hunt, C. R., "Proto-oncogene mRNA Levels and Activities of Multiple Transcription Factors in C3H 10T 1/2 Murine Embryonic Fibroblasts

Over 50 different proto-oncogenes are at work in the human body. They function as receptors and signalers for growth factors that stimulate the production of numerous essential proteins. Alteration of proto-oncogene activity can lead to mutations that convert normal proto-oncogenes into abnormal oncogenes. Since proto-oncogenes promote cell division, once they are mutated into oncogenes, they similarly promote abnormal cell division. Excessive cellular proliferation of this type promotes rapid cancer growth.[216]

Cellular Calcium Ions Modified

EMR, across the spectrum, alters calcium ion homeostasis in cells. Calcium is vital in normal cell functioning and survival. Calcium ions are extremely important, because they initiate several of the bodily functions discussed in previous chapters. They play a fundamental role in regulating the GABA neurotransmitter, melatonin production, DNA synthesis, cell death, chromosome aberrations, gene transcription, protein expression, immune system competence, heart rhythm, reproduction, and the nervous system.

Since calcium ions have so many essential responsibilities, calcium efflux in cells can wreak havoc on the body by imposing a wide variety of adverse health effects in any one or more of the previously mentioned areas.

Stress Response Enhanced

The cells of nearly every life form on earth respond to environmental attacks similarly. When life-threatening danger is sensed, they resort to a mode of protection and self-preservation. This survival "stress response" produces stress proteins, also known as heat shock proteins. Numerous environmental hazards, such as toxins, chemicals, lack of oxygen, and extreme heat, cause cells to respond in this manner. Scientists have discovered that cells behave in this same fashion when they are exposed to low levels of ELF and RF. An increase in the molecular stress response has been observed in cells immediately following cell phone exposure.[217]

Exposed to 835.62 and 847.74 MHz Cellular Telephone Communication Frequency Radiation," *Radiat Res* Vol. 151 No. 3 (1999): pp. 300-309.

[216] Raven, Johnson, Losos, and Singer, *Biology, 7th Edition*, (New York, NY: McGraw Hill, 2005). p.416.

[217] Lai, Henry, *"Biological Effects of Radiofrequency Radiation"*, Paper for the Scientific Workshop "EMF-Scientific and Legal Issues, Theory and Evidence of EMF Biological and Health Effects" in Catania, Sicily, Italy, September 13-14,

When normal proteins turn into heat shock proteins, they are altered and can eventually lose their defensive function. Even at levels considered safe by U.S. standard setters, RF/MW radiation induces the development of irregular heat shock proteins. This repeated response can cause cells to become cancerous.[218]

Dr. Peter French of the Centre for Immunology, St. Vincent's Hospital in Sydney, Australia, has led multiple experiments on both human and animal cell lines to uncover their responses to cell phone radiation. French and his team validated the fact that exposure to mobile phone radiation can elicit cancer. This conclusion was derived at after observing that repeated mobile phone use induces the chronic production of heat shock proteins without significantly generating heat. The increase of heat shock proteins elevates the risk of tumor and cancer development, speeds metastasis (the spread of cancer cells by way of the blood stream), and decreases the effectiveness of anti-cancer drugs.[219]

Significant Promotion of Multiple Cancers

Significant dose-response relationships have repeatedly been shown to exist between RF/MW radiation exposure and all types of cancer. Multiple research efforts show that brain tumors, leukemia, and lymphoma are especially RF sensitive.[220] Evidence of these occurrences has been demonstrated at current residential exposure levels, those which are presumably safe by U.S. government standards.[221] In other words, cell phone users aren't the only ones being affected. Reports also confirm that increases in total mortality rate exist from these exposure-induced cancers.

2002, organized by the Italian National Institute for Prevention and Work Safety. [De Pomerai et al. (2000, 2002)].

[218] Maisch, Don, "Mobile Phone Use: it's time to take precautions," *Journal of the Australasian College of Nutritional and Environmental Medicine*, Vol. 20, No. 1, April 2001.

[219] Melbourne, Alan, "Problems with the Rationale of the Draft Standard", http://www.ssec.org.au/emraa/rf/may.htm (May 11, 2001).

[220] Cherry, Neil *"Evidence that Electromagnetic Radiation is Genotoxic: The Implications for the Epidemiology of Cancer and Cardiac, Neurological and Reproductive Effects,"* Extended from a paper presented to the conference on Possible Health Effects on Health of Radiofrequency Electromagnetic Fields, 29th June 2000, European Parliament, Brussels. p.44

[221] Cherry, Neil, "Health Effects Associated with Mobile Base Stations in Communities: the need for health studies," http://www.mapcruzin.com/radiofrequency/cherry/neil_cherry1.htm (June 8, 2000).

Although no adequate long term studies have been conducted on cell phone users and cancer, because consumer use is still considered somewhat short term, Australian studies on laboratory animals have revealed some insightful information. Mice exposed to cell phone radiation for 9-18 months developed twice as many tumors as those who weren't.[222] Other scientists found that 18 irradiated rats developed malignant tumors from exposure as compared to only 5 rats in the unexposed control group.[223]

Prompted by former statistics and a Swedish study conducted in 2000, confirming evidence of increased brain tumor risk on the side of the head where cell phones are held, the World Health Organization (WHO) requested that a multi-national study on the subject be conducted. Dr. Lennart Hardell, from the Oncology Department at Orebro, in Sweden, headed the effort.

From the WHO recommended follow-up study, Hardell was able to reconfirm and validate conclusions from other previous research efforts. Across the board it was determined that cell phone users do have a greater risk of developing a brain tumor on the same side of the head that the handset is held, than on the opposite side, where exposure is not as intense. According to the study, the risk was 2.4 times greater, thus, restituting the fact that cell phone use does cause cancer. [224]

To address the global uncertainty of this relationship between cell phone use and brain tumor development, 14 scientists, public health officials, and public policy experts composed the BioInitiative Report. This report was a concentrated effort to extract and interpret all available, pertinent data gathered from years of research and multiple worldwide studies. The extensive, in depth undertaking revealed that cell phone users of 10+ years are without a doubt posed with a higher risk of developing brain tumors as well as acoustic neuromas. However, the increased threat varies depending on how the phone is used. If you alternate head sides while talking on your cell phone, there is a 20% danger of developing a brain

---

[222] Fist, Stewart, "Cell Phones and Cancer," *The Australian Newspaper*, May 5, 1997.

[223] Foster K. R. and Guy, A. W., "The Microwave Problem," Scientific American Vol. 255, No. 3 (September 1986): pp. 32-39.

[224] George Carlo and Martin Schram, *Cell Phones: Invisible Hazards of the Wireless Age* (New York, NY: Carroll & Graf Publishers, 2001), pp. 168-177.

tumor. Conversely, if you don't rotate sides, your brain tumor risk increases to 200%. [225]

Leukemia

Residential studies, focusing on the effects of RF/MW radiation from cell towers, have been performed throughout the world and every study has found a significant increase in both adult and childhood leukemia in exposed populations. Leukemia mortality rates were also higher. [226] Research efforts have revealed that every one who works, resides, or spends a large majority of time within five miles of a site is adversely affected. Those residing closest to the radiating antennas are exposed to the strongest signals, thereby experiencing the greatest detriment. Distance reduces risk.

Children are much more susceptible to microwaves than adults; therefore their risk of developing leukemia is much higher. In an effort to conceal the accuracy of incriminating findings, which have consistently shown elevated levels of childhood leukemia as a result of various RF exposures, studies bought and performed by interested parties, who benefit from a "no effect" result, have recruited older children as participants. Since younger children are more vulnerable to the effects of radiation, operating in this manner skews the outcome so risk levels do not reach "statistical significance". In doing this, the results are more acceptable to everyone: those funding the study, the researchers, and the general public.

Acoustic Neuroma

Acoustic neuroma is a rare, non-cancerous tumor that impairs the hearing nerve. Documented cases are becoming more common and rates have continued to rise in conjunction with the use of cell phones. Those who have been using a cell phone for 3+ years have a 30%-60% chance of acquiring acoustic neuroma. [227] Further, if

---

[225] Sage, C., *The Bio Initiative Report,*
http://www.bioinitiative.org/report/docs/section_1.pdf (May 2008), p. 9.
[226] Cherry, Neil *"Evidence that Electromagnetic Radiation is Genotoxic: The Implications for the Epidemiology of Cancer and Cardiac, Neurological and Reproductive Effects,"* Extended from a paper presented to the conference on Possible Health Effects on Health of Radiofrequency Electromagnetic Fields, 29th June 2000, European Parliament, Brussels. pp. 36-37.
[227] George Carlo and Martin Schram, *Cell Phones: Invisible Hazards of the Wireless Age* (New York, NY: Carroll & Graf Publishers, 2001), p. 170.

a cell phone is used primarily on one side of the head, the risk increases to 240%. For cordless phones, the risk is 310%.

Rapid Cancer Growth

It has been established through a number of studies that the cell proliferation of mutated oncogenes from cell phone radiation, accelerates cancer growth.[228]

Drs. Czerska, Casamento, Ning, and Davis of the FDA, observed the rapid multiplication of human cancer cells when they were exposed to a waveform identical to that used in digital cellular phones.[229]

Further evidence supporting this phenomenon, revealed that radio waves from mobile handsets not only cause cancerous cells to grow at an unusually fast rate, aggressive cell proliferation continues even after exposure has stopped.

Russian and Italian researchers have arrived at this astonishing conclusion that "a few minutes of exposure to cell phone type radiation can transform a 5% tumor into a 95% active cancer!"[230]

Deceptive Studies

Uncertainty and controversy continue to test the link between cell phone use and cancer. On one hand you have leading research experts who have, independently from each other, proven that cell phone radiation causes DNA damage. Evidence of this damage, represented by micronuclei in exposed human blood cells, is an unmistakable diagnostic indicator used by medical professionals to determine if a patient is posed with a high risk of developing cancer or tumors. On the other hand, you have studies proving no effect. Let's take a closer look.

Between 1982 and 1995, one of the biggest cancer studies was conducted. Over 420,000 Danish mobile phone users participated; of those, the majority had only been using their phone for three years and only several thousand had over ten years of use.

---

[228] Raven, Johnson, Losos, and Singer, *Biology, 7th Edition*, (New York, NY: McGraw Hill, 2005), p.416.

[229] E.M. Czerska, J. Casamento, J. T. Ning, and C. Davis, *"Effects of Radiofrequency Electromagnetic Radiation on Cell Proliferation,"* Abstract presented on February 7, 1997 at the workshop 'Physical Characteristics and Possible Biological Effects of Microwaves Applied in Wireless Communication, Rockville, MD.

[230] Woollhams, C., "Are Mobiles a Health Hazard?", *Police Magazine,* December 2002.

While this long term study appeared to be legit, it was deceptive. Being fully aware that it normally takes more than ten years for cancer to develop, the outcome of this industry-funded study was highly predictable. It boasted of showing no adverse health effects or cancer development. When the exciting news of "no cancer risk from cell phone use" was disclosed to the world, the critical data of having based their study on short term usage was never mentioned.

Likewise, other seemingly valid studies, performed by credible sources, have been based on short term usage and therefore report no cancer risk. Two U.S. epidemiological efforts fall into this category. The first was conducted in 2001 by the National Cancer Institute and the second was conducted by the American Health Foundation.

The National Cancer Institute reported no significant increase in brain tumor after reviewing 782 brain tumor cases. However, of these, only 52 had used a mobile phone for over 3 years and only 35 of them confessed to having been on their phone for more than 15 minutes a day.

Joshua Muscat, who led the study for the American Health Foundation, claimed that, "the data showed no correlation between the use of cell phones and the development of brain cancer". What he didn't expose was that of the 469 brain tumor cases, the average cell phone usage was 2.8 years.

As you can see, although these findings are being reported by reliable sources, the basis upon which they are making their claims are not only irrelevant, they're unreasonable and deceptive.[231]

---

[231] Maisch, Don, "Mobile Phone Use: it's time to take precautions, 2001. Reprinted from *Journal of the Australasian College of Nutritional and Environmental Medicine,* Vol. 20, No. 1, April 2001.

CHAPTER 10

Tower Trauma

After learning that a direct correlation exists between RF/MW radiation and all types of cancer at current residential exposure levels, it becomes apparent that the sources emitting this harmful energy into our environment are making people sick. Not only are there increases in cancer because of this carcinogenic irritant, all of the symptoms of Microwave Sickness are similarly escalating. Unfortunately, whether you're a cell phone user or not, you are under attack; constantly being bombarded by RF/MW radiation emissions from cell towers, their sites, and antennas. There are so many of these radiating apparatuses, that it's virtually impossible to run or hide from their microwave signals.

Due to the vast number of these signaling masts and their counterparts (lobes and panels which are attached to the top of buildings, water towers, etc.), emissions radiate through every body within signal range. In other words, every person within a 5-mile radius of the source, or in the same range of multiple sources, is chronically being irradiated, 24 hours a day, 7 days a week, and 365 days a year. However, cell phone users endure a more intense assault when their wireless device is "on", because not only is their body responding to the involuntary irradiation of nearby signals, increased doses of microwaves are constantly being transmitted between your phone and your service provider's nearest base station.

Tower emissions in the U.S. are higher than any where else in the world, with the exception of the United Kingdom. For example, U.S. towers are allowed to emit 5800 times more RF/MW radiation than similar base stations in Salzburg, Austria. [232] Now that's a point to ponder. If Austria's towers serve the same fundamental purpose at significantly reduced levels of radiation, then why are Americans being exposed to so much more radiation?

Microwaves from cell towers affect us in much the same way as those from cell phones. The only difference is that the RF/MW radiation from cell sites is absorbed by the entire body rather than being concentrated and focused directly at your head. And although the tower's signal strength is substantially stronger than the signal strength from your cell phone, the non-ionizing radiation absorbed into the body as a whole, can more easily and effectively dissipate the deep tissue heating effect which results from this type of exposure. While cell phone operators seem to be willing to accept some degree of undisclosed risk in regards to their wireless communication decisions, those residing or working in close proximity to cell towers are not so privileged. Since the majority of people remain entirely unaware of any health related risks associated with these unsightly monstrosities, they cannot exercise any options relating to exposure. Instead, they stand idly by being irradiated.

Cellular communication tower sites are strategically placed within five miles of one another. While initially this may not sound like it would equate to many towers, it does when you consider that every single service provider in the area has to have its own network. In large metropolitan areas there can be several service providers, and with each needing its own network, that adds up to a lot of towers. Additionally, each network has to position its towers within communication range and line of site of each other in every direction. It's seriously disturbing when you begin to realize the tremendous number of cell sites you are being impacted by in the areas where you live, work, and play.

The good news about cell towers being placed close together is that they don't need to transmit as much energy as towers which are farther apart. Reduced power means that absorption potential is also lessened. The bad news is that, in order for numerous service providers to accomplish the goal of a 5-mile radius, towers must be placed in close proximity of one another or site owners can lease space on the site they are currently using to competing providers. Evidence of service provider cooperation can be observed whenever

---

[232] Brown, Gary, *Wireless Devices, Standards, and Microwave Radiation in the Education Environment,* http://www.emfacts.com/wlans.html, (October 2000).

134

you see multiple levels of omni-directional transceivers in the form of panels, cones, drums, lobes, or antennas circling the top of tower structures. Additional signal facilitators increase exposure as well as absorption potential.

Tower Exposure Studies

Universally, via numerous global studies, conducted by multiple independent researchers and governments, two very important facts have repeatedly been confirmed. The first is that RF/MW radiation emissions from cell towers around the world exhibit a consistent and very significant dose-response relationship between dozens of neurological symptoms and cancer development. Health problems and complaints, which precede cancer, are inevitable as they escalate in occurrence and severity over time in residents living near cell towers. Comparisons made between cell site radiation exposure patterns and residential cancer patterns systematically correlated, proving that higher cancer rates exist in residents living closest to cell towers. Mortality rates have also been shown to be extremely significant; more than a doubling of natural numbers.

The second confirmed fact is that those who live closest to the radiating sites are posed with the greatest threat. The farther you reside from a cell tower, the safer you are. Distance has continually proven to be the one determining factor between residential levels of exposure and health risk.

After studying a compilation of multiple residential epidemiology studies, research expert Dr. Neil Cherry made some presumptions about the unwavering results. "Cell sites will probably acutely increase miscarriage, depression, suicide, sleep disturbance, and chronically increase rates of cancer, many diseases, significant neurological and cardiac diseases and death." He goes on to say, "The problems are going to increase unless rapid, drastic and determined moves are made to reverse the trend and only install new sites in locations that produce extremely low mean residential exposures."[233]

---

[233] Cherry, Neil *"Evidence that Electromagnetic Radiation is Genotoxic: The Implications for the Epidemiology of Cancer and Cardiac, Neurological and Reproductive Effects,"* Extended from a paper presented to the conference on Possible Health Effects on Health of Radiofrequency Electromagnetic Fields, 29th June 2000, European Parliament, Brussels. p. 56.

Over the past 5+ years, as concern surrounding these questionable radiating devices has escalated, residents of various communities have tried to fight the erection of cell towers around their homes. Although admirable, such efforts remain unsuccessful because of the 1996 Telecommunications Act.

The 1996 Telecommunications Act

In order to overcome potential problems that could interrupt the steady and rapid erection of cell towers throughout the nation, the cellular industry established the 1996 Telecommunications Act. This act became law on February 8, 1996. It was devised to significantly restrict the ability of local communities, authorities, and residents to resist the placement of cell towers, especially where health related issues were concerned.

As you recall, the U.S. Government does not govern the cell phone industry, the industry governs itself. Therefore it possesses the same rights and freedoms as utility companies. Service providers can place and position their cell towers and counterparts wherever they want them, without restriction, except on private property where a contractual agreement for lease does not exist. The industry is also its own final authority and even though they are supposed to abide by set guidelines, the FCC has admitted that it simply doesn't have the manpower to police all of their efforts. Instead, the government empowers and trusts the cellular industry to conduct its own monitoring of tower and phone emission levels.

The Act also limits the FCC's power to intervene when local communities or authorities object to tower placement. Instead of listening to or effectively addressing legitimate concerns, the service provider pacifies disgruntled residents by allowing them to choose from a number of tower construction options.[234] In doing this, they can eliminate the "eye sore" issue, but little else.

In order to mask their identity, cell towers are being hidden on rooftops and above water towers; they are being discreetly housed inside flag poles, church steeples, bell towers, crosses, silos, and clock towers. They are also being concealed in road signs, commercial signs, telephone poles, and billboards. Cell towers are even made to resemble and blend in with the tall pines of Northern

---

[234] Kipp, Vicki. (May 2001). *"Tower Industry Part 5 – Tower Location,"* Society of Broadcast Engineers Newsletter.

California, the palm trees of Southern California, and the Giant Saguaro cactuses of Arizona. There is virtually no limit as to how these cell sites are being hidden and disguised.

In an effort to establish just how effective the Telecommunications Act is, allow me to share another personal experience. Due to his long term exposure, my late husband Steve, like hundreds of thousands of other normal, healthy people worldwide, had developed a relentless sensitivity to EMR and RF energy.

After finally connecting his numerous symptoms and the development of brain damage to Steve's occupational exposure of RF/MW radiation, we realized the debilitating impact that the emanating microwaves from nearby cell towers had on him and we were deeply concerned. He had such a heightened sensitivity to that type of energy that whenever he was in close proximity of a site for more than twenty minutes, his face would turn bright red, he would become extremely irritable, and his thought and communication processes would completely shut down. At that time, he was unable to comprehend that which was being said and he was unable to respond. Episodes like these, of such intense exposure, would keep him bedridden for days. I was extremely thankful that we lived in a fairly remote area where nearby exposure was minimal.

One afternoon at a local post office I was talking with the postmaster about Steve's condition and his odd response to cell towers. She was familiar with and empathetic to our situation. On that day she regrettably gave me some very upsetting news; she told me that the owner of the property on which the post office sat, had signed a contract with AT&T to lease them space for a cell tower. The pending location was just a stone's throw away from our newly constructed, custom designed home. I was speechless and inquired further for definite confirmation. I knew that if what she was telling me was true, little could be done to change the inevitable, based on the 1996 Telecommunications Act.

Not wanting to believe what I had just heard, with tears streaming down my face I raced over to the township office. Before reaching the door I struggled to contain my obvious state of distress. Inside I spoke with the zoning administrator, Ms. James. I shared with her what I had just been informed of. She had heard nothing about the agreement and proceeded to assure me that a tower would never be erected in that location even if such a contract did exist. Reason being, that the property was zoned for residential use and was not in an area where a cell tower could be placed. I challenged her beliefs, stating that my research had led me to conclude otherwise and that her convictions simply weren't true. But, she like many others didn't accept that which I was telling her.

Being fully aware of how upset I was, she again confidentially assured me that no such union would ever take place in the designated location. As I walked out the door I knew she was wrong.

Upon returning home I conferred with Steve. Because of our understanding of the 1996 Telecommunications Act, we realized the perilous predicament we were in. We both knew that we had to act and act fast. There was no time to waste; we had no choice, but to move. We didn't want to move again; we had no where to go. We wanted to stay in our new house near family and friends; we wanted our children to remain in the same school with their friends. The timing wasn't right, four years earlier we had moved from across the nation, but because of Steve's sensitivity, we knew staying was not an option.

Just 6 months after finding a very remote safe haven for Steve, the girls and I returned to visit family and friends. I was eager to drive by our former house; it was truly no surprise to see a cell tower right where the postmaster said it would be, less than ¼ mile away. With a calm and curious demeanor, I paid another visit to the township zoning administrator. I asked Ms. James if she remembered me and our past conversation. She did. I asked her what had happened with the tower that now stands where she promised it never would. Defensively, she told me that the township and numerous people of the community fought the good fight, but when all was said and done, the battle was lost.

Ms. James confessed that she was surprised by the amount of authority that has been given to the industry to do whatever it is they want to do. Their disregard to the zoning laws and their immunity from having to comply with them came as a shock. Only by having extremely strong zoning laws established and local government authorities who are willing to do what it takes to go up against the multi-billion dollar industry can placement be diverted. These instances are rare. Outside of that, nothing can be done to stop the rapid expansion and development of the wireless networks that continue to grow in our residential neighborhoods and communities.

Cell Tower Placement

Because undeniable proof of increased vulnerability in children, the sick, the weak, and the elderly to RF/MW radiation exposure, some countries prohibit the placement of cell towers and antennas near schools, daycares, hospitals, and nursing homes. However, here in the U.S., these sites are often prime locations for tower placement.

Schools are an easy target for service providers, because they are always in such desperate need of revenue. School administrators are constantly seeking ways to make ends meet. They're willing to consider just about anything to get their needs met, including placing cell towers on top of the school or on school property. This usually provides a very lucrative stream of monthly income, which can continue for years, depending on the contractual agreement. Nevertheless, the seemingly worthwhile exchange of space for facility upgrades, books, playground equipment, computers, and the like has a bigger price tag than most would ever suspect.

Additionally, installing Wi-Fi systems into the schools or homes where children endure chronic, long term exposure is not a decision that should be taken lightly. These microwaves operate at higher frequencies than cell phones, potentially increasing the threat of harm. Children are much more vulnerable to their effects than adults because their bodies are smaller, much easier to infiltrate, and they absorb more radiation at a faster rate.

Numerous research efforts have indicated that children exposed to this type of wireless radiation are affected in a variety of ways; none of which are positive. There has been repeated evidence of significantly slowed reaction times, reduced memory capacity, learning impairments, concentration difficulties, altered brain waves which leads to behavior changes and mood swings, cognitive and motor skill dysfunction, and immune system irregularities.[235]

It is extremely worrisome that such a desirable technological device which offers numerous benefits can cause so many adverse health effects, especially in our youth.

---

[235] Chiang, H. Yao, G. D., Fang, Q. S., Wang K. Q., Lu, D. Z. and Zhou, Y. K., "Health Effects of Environmental Electromagnetic Fields," *J. Bioelectricity,* 1989, volume 8, pp. 127-131.

Firefighters Fight Back

Over the past several years, there has been growing concern among U.S. and Canadian firefighters, regarding the placement of cell towers on the rooftops of fire stations. As with schools, when it comes to positioning towers, wireless service providers target municipal buildings. Fire stations are also considered key locations, because of their centralized locations and the fact that the industry can avoid any unnecessary red tape. Local authorities receive tremendous compensation from such contractual arrangements, benefiting handsomely from each and every tower placed on all city, county, state, or government owned properties, including fire stations, schools, and the like.

In August of 2004, the issue was formerly addressed at the International Association of Fire Fighters (IAFF) Convention in Boston, MA. There, Lt. Ron Cronin of the Brookline, MA, Fire Department openly expressed concern. "Some firefighters with cell towers currently located on their stations are experiencing symptoms that put our first responders at risk. It is important to be sure we understand what effects these towers may have on the firefighters living in these stations. If the jakes in the fire houses are suffering from headaches, can't respond quickly and their ability to make decisions is clouded by a sort of brain fog, then entire communities they are protecting will clearly be at risk. No one wants the guys responding to their family emergency to be functioning at anything less than 100 percent capacity."

Cronin's statement was in response to a study of firefighters who had been residing in stations with rooftop tower antennas for up to five years. It was found that they suffered from similar neurological abnormalities as those who suffer from Microwave Sickness: slowed reaction time, lack of focus, lack of impulse control, severe headaches, anesthesia-like sleep, sleep deprivation, depression, and tremors. Individual brain scans also revealed mutual gross irregularities.[236]

---

[236] *International Association of Fire Fighters, AFL-CIO, CLC,* Division of Occupational Health, Safety, and Medicine. http://www.iaff.org/hs/resi/celltowerfinal.htm (March 2005). Concerns of cell tower placement on fire stations was brought forth at the International Association of Fire Fighters (IAFF) convention, Boston, MA August 2004.

In 1995 a retired couple bought a resort home east of Vancover, B.C. Both enjoyed good health until they claimed that their world came crashing down. What began with buzzing sounds in the distance, led to uncomfortable pressure in the head and ears. The symptoms were followed by severe headache, neck and shoulder pain, and continual nausea that increased with time. Relief was found only when the couple traveled 30 minutes away from their home. One year after moving into their dream home, the man became so ill that he and his wife had to leave. The incident destroyed their golden years, along with their marriage.

Through his personal research, the man discovered that he was being affected by the radiation of a nearby cell tower. He made the following statement, "I would advise anyone that lives near a tower and starts to feel the following symptoms to move fast before you become sensitive as I have. The symptoms started with a buzzing sound and developed into a high pitch sizzle sound in my head, pressure headaches, blocked ears, pain in neck, shoulder and other joints, nausea, stress, burning eyes, fuzzy vision, memory loss, imbalance and fatigue."

Another senior citizen describes moving into a 20th floor apartment of a government subsidized housing facility. "I immediately began experiencing symptoms of a dizzy, off balance feeling, headaches which were constant, severe insomnia, profuse nose bleeds, …I wasn't able to concentrate. I would often find myself…feeling "out of it", not remembering. I felt drained…I had anxiety attacks and breathlessness, felt agitated, restless and my joints and my eyes were sore. My chest felt pressure."

A magazine article disclosed to this apartment resident that microwaves from cell towers emit harmful radiation that impacts humans in much the same ways as he had been experiencing. He began to pay close attention to his surroundings and discovered that the rooftop of his complex, just one floor above where he resided, housed at least 25 telecommunication antennas and microwave towers. He proclaimed, "The top of the building looks like a porcupine!"[237]

---

[237] Riedlinger, Robert, "Electro-magnetic Emissions Enough to Make Some People Sick", *Citizens Initiative Omega*, Vol. 24, No. 06, 2003.

Sheila Rogers, editor of Latitudes, a quarterly publication of the Association for Comprehensive NeuroTherapy shared a despairing story of two dairy farmers and how a nearby cell tower affected their family. A 150 acre parcel of land and a farming business had been passed down through the generations to Meredith, her husband, and their four children. Soon after its acquisition, a neighbor had a cell tower erected on his property, 800 feet from the farmer's happy home. Although unsightly, they were assured that the tower was completely safe.

Over the next six months, the herd that grazed near the tower became discontented and easily agitated; their hides became tough. All four children developed unusual, raised skin rashes and experienced recurring kidney infections. The two younger children became dramatically hyperactive, while the older two complained of foggy thinking and concentration difficulties. Sleep disturbances affected the entire family and Meredith, in her early thirties, suffered from joint problems.

While searching for answers, the writer says, "They tracked down a researcher at the EPA. He told Meredith that as a government official he should reassure her that they (cell towers) were safe." He proceeded to follow that with a strict warning, "But with his 'citizen cap' on, he had to say that they should move immediately".

After selling the herd and moving to an area away from cell towers in Michigan's Upper Peninsula, everyone's symptoms subsided. Within one year they regained their strength and were ready to return to the farm. The family was reassured by the cell phone company that the tower was absolutely safe.

Following their return, problems began to resurface. The children lost weight and their hair was falling out. Meredith gave birth to a son born with birth defects the doctor couldn't explain. The neighbors were also experiencing unusual complications. Town residents were seeing an increased rate of suicide and abnormal seizure activity. Even the new herd of cattle exhibited abnormalities. Calves were being born with front legs shorter than the back ones, their hooves were deformed, they were no longer chewing their cud, and unusual tumors developed.

After moving away from the situation, the writer asked Meredith, "What happened to the farm? Meredith sighs, 'It just sits there. Empty. Selling the farm has not been considered. Should we let this happen to someone else?'"

Such stories, while seemingly rare, are not as uncommon as you may think. I have heard similar stories from numerous people. Purely coincidence? I highly doubt it.

Electro-sensitive people in this country are often scoffed at and challenged. Their circumstances make it difficult for them to function, let alone drive, hold a job, or maintain relationships. Even with assistance, it is a financial strain to fund all the prescription drugs that are supposed to offer relief. It's really a shame because ultimately these people can truly become imprisoned, socially, physically, and environmentally.

Different Cell Tower Variations

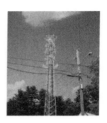

Most Common Cell Towers

The number and levels of antennas and panels give evidence that these sites are shared by multiple service providers.

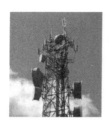

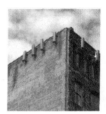

Microwave Communication Panels on Buildings

In metropolitan areas where tower space is limited, service providers lease panel space on sides of buildings and rooftops.

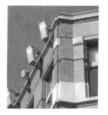

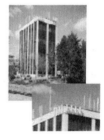

Cell Cites, Antennas, and Satellite Dishes Top Buildings

Numerous buildings across the nation, especially municipal and hospital buildings, lease rooftop space to service providers.

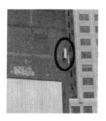

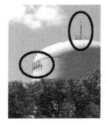

Communication Panels Can Be Placed Anywhere

Water towers, smoke stacks, or any place that offers the height necessary to transmit signals serve as desirable locations for placement.

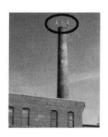

More Cell Towers

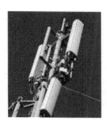

Flat, Semi-Rounded Panels and Single Antenna Lobes

These types of microwave transmitters and receivers offer numerous placement options, including atop telephone poles.

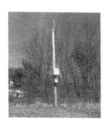

Rod-Shaped Masts

Such masts are easily disguised in a variety of ways. Some of the most common hiding places are inside flag poles, crosses, and other tall cylinder-like entities.

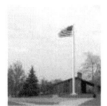

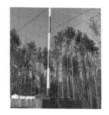

Cell Sites are Everywhere

With such versatility, microwave signals can be transmitted and received from just about anywhere.
There are few exceptions.

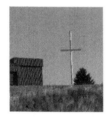

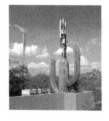

Natural Beauty or Cell Site?

Cell towers are becoming commonplace in our natural environment. You can see their communication panels hidden in cactuses, palm trees, and pine trees.

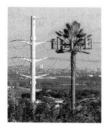

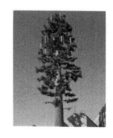

CHAPTER 11

The Consequential Impact on Our Youth

Children and teens are the fastest growing group of mobile phone users in the world. Coincidentally, they are also the most vulnerable to the hazards associated with its exposure. What's worse is that with full knowledge of what worldwide studies have shown regarding this incompatible union, the industry continues to heavily promote their phones to our the youth with explicit intent and with clear, direct messages. Over the past several years the industry has successfully been able to convince the younger generation that it is socially unacceptable not to have a cell phone.

Scientists, researchers, experts, and medical professionals from around the world who are familiar with RF/MW radiation and the adverse health effects linked to cell phone use, are strongly discouraging young people from using cell phones. There are 5 principal reasons why children are so much more susceptible to this type of intrusive external stimuli than adults:

1) Children have thinner skulls, making it easier for cell phone RF/MW radiation to penetrate;
2) the rapid division of cells in children dramatically increases their risk of DNA damage;
3) children have underdeveloped immune systems which are not equipped to protect them from this harmful carcinogen;[238]

---

[238] *Health Effects of Microwave Radiation (Western View),*
http://www.goodhealthinfo.net/radiation/health_efx_western.htm (March 2007).

4) the young brains of children absorb close to 50% more radiation; and [239]
5) children's brains and eyes absorb microwaves at a rate of 3.3 times faster.

In 1996, Dr. Om Gandhi, a widely respected scientist from the University of Utah, released a warning regarding children and cell phone use. His study concluded that while pressing the operating device against the head, the amount of microwave radiation measured in milliwatts per kilogram (mW/kg) being absorbed into an adult brain is approximately 7.84; in a ten year old child the absorption rate escalates to 19.77; in a five year old child the level of absorbed radiation sky rockets to a frightening 33.12! Research has shown that doses of less than 5 mW/kg produce enough deep tissue heating to cause damage to the human brain.[240]

Along with these astonishing absorption rates, it was observed that younger children with the thinnest skulls have the most sensitive brain tissue; therefore they incur a greater degree of injury. Since the smallest of children are posed with the greatest threat, it goes without saying that infants are at maximum risk. This data establishes the fact that when it comes to absorption, not only is a child's delicate body significantly weaker than an adult's, but their underdeveloped immune system lacks the ability to fight against an assault of RF/MW energy, thus leaving them defenseless. In other words, due to this reality, children are much more prone to the development of genetic damage and other related adverse health effects.[241]

Altered Brain Waves, Altered Behavior

Dr. Michael Klieeisen of the Neuro Diagnostic Research Institute in Marbella, Spain, has ascertained from his research that after a child is exposed to the cell phone radiation from just one short call, he experiences a significant slowing and altering of brain

---

[239] C.H. Durney, *et al.,* "An Empirical Formula for Broad-Band SAR Calculations of Prolate Spheroidal Models of Humans and Animals," *IEEE Transactions on Microwave Theory and Techniques* MTT-27, No. 8 (August 1979): pp. 758-763.
[240] Robert Kane, *Cellular Telephone Russian Roulette* (New York, NY: Vantage Press, 2001), p. 45.
[241] George Carlo and Martin Schram, *Cell Phones: Invisible Hazards of the Wireless Age* (New York, NY: Carroll & Graf Publishers, 2001), pp. 215-217.

function.[242] Like Klieeisen, Dr. Gerard Hyland, a physicist at Warwick University, Coventry, England, examined brain wave changes in children following short mobile phone calls. Hyland's comment regarding his research is painstakingly insightful. "The results show that children's brains are affected for long periods even after very short-term use. Their brain wave patterns are abnormal and stay like that for a long period. This could affect their mood and ability to learn ... Alteration in brain waves could lead to...lack of concentration, memory loss, inability to learn and aggressive behavior."

Based on the results of his findings, Hyland offers this admonition, "If I were a parent I would now be extremely wary about allowing my children to use a mobile even for a very short period. My advice would be to avoid mobiles."[243]

Teen Brain Damage

Dr. Lief Salford, a neurosurgeon at Lund University in Sweden, published author, and respected researcher of multiple RF/MW radiation studies, and his colleagues conducted studies on GSM (digital) cell phone radiation to establish its effects on teenagers. Salford tested rats between 12-26 weeks old because they are the same developmental age of human teenagers. The rodents were exposed to two hours of microwave radiation and fifty days later there was "highly significant evidence" of brain damage throughout the cranium.[244]

It was also discovered that neuronal damage increased in accordance with exposure; a definite indication of a clear dose-response relationship. Salford noted, "If this effect was to transfer to young mobile users, the effects could be terrifying. We can see

---

[242] Woollhams, C., "Are Mobiles a Health Hazard?", *Police Magazine,* December 2002.
[243] ACN Online, "Electrical Sensitivity: A Global Growing Concern. How Wireless Technology May Impact Child Development and Central Nervous System Functioning," Association for Comprehensive Neurotherapy.
[244] BBC News Health Contents: Medical Notes, February 5, 2003, "Mobile Phones May Trigger Alzheimer's," http://news.bbc.co.uk/2/low/health/2728149.stm

reduced brain capacity, meaning those who might normally have got Alzheimer's dementia in old age could get in much earlier."[245]

As previously mentioned, an article recently published in one of the nation's top newspapers reported that our society is beginning to see a considerable influx of people under the age of forty being diagnosed with Alzheimer's disease. This fatal and destructive disease, which used to be restricted to those with an inherited genetic link and to the elderly, is now swiftly merging into younger populations and affecting those with no family history of the ailment. Although the article offered no rationale for the mounting menace, we can only presuppose that since RF/MW radiation exposure has repeatedly been shown to lead to the development of Alzheimer's and other neurodegenerative diseases, it is highly possible that the root cause could be attributed to the rapid acceleration of this environmental carcinogen.

Following his study, Dr. Salford appeared on the UK BCC radio program "You and Yours", which was broadcast on February 5, 2003. As a concerned scientist and father, Salford took full advantage of the opportunity he was given to educate his audience. Based on his research findings, Salford had become thoroughly convinced that brain damage from cell phone use is a "probability rather than a possibility", more likely than not to develop. He also stated publicly that he would not allow his children to use a mobile phone for any reason outside of an emergency. Salford also reported that he was no longer willing to use his mobile unless it was for something important.[246]

Global Warnings to Parents

One critical fact that cannot be overlooked when discussing this topic is that our youth are starting to use cell phones at a much younger age than first generation cell phone users. This long term exposure significantly elevates their risk of consequences. Not only are our children more likely to develop adverse health effects they are more likely to develop them at a much younger age.

---

[245] ACN Online, "Electrical Sensitivity: A Global Growing Concern. How Wireless Technology May Impact Child Development and Central Nervous System Functioning," Association for Comprehensive Neurotherapy.

[246] "Mobile Phone Signals Kill Brain Cells", http://www.powerwatch.org.uk/ (February 6, 2003).

With the realization of this truth, along with available research data, it is no wonder that experts and professional organizations from around the world are making an unwavering stand against children using cell phones. The following list identifies a number of associations, governments, and individuals who feel that there is an urgently pressing need to educate parents and warn the public about the grave dangers we put our youth in when we place a cell phone in their hands.

- **The San Francisco Medical Society**

  The San Francisco Medical Society has advised parents that even, "The use of 'kiddy mobile phones'…are terrible ideas at this point".[247]

- **The German Academy of Pediatrics**

  The German Academy of Pediatrics has issued a statement advising parents to restrict their children's cell phone use. They strongly discourage against the unnecessary, frequent and extended use of mobiles by children. In addition, the Academy called for stricter RF/MW exposure limits and advised that all mobile phone users keep their calls as "brief as possible". [248, 249]

- **The Federal Authority for Radiation Protection in Germany**

  Wolfram Koenig, head of the Federal Authority for Radiation Protection in Germany, stated in an interview that, "Parents should take their children away from that technology [mobile phones]." He also urged the industry not to target children in their advertising campaigns.[250]

---

[247] *San Francisco Medical Society,* http://www.sfms.org/sfm/sfm301h.htm (2007).

[248] German Academy of Pediatrics: Keep Kids Away From Mobiles," *Microwave News* Vol. 21, No. 4 (Jan/Feb 2001): p. 5.

[249] Maisch, , Don, "Mobile Phone Use: It's Time to Take Precautions," *ACNEM Journal,* Vol. 20, No. 1, (April 2001): p. 4.

[250] *Berliner Morgenpost,* July 31, 2001.

- ## German Medical Doctors of the Interdisciplinary Association for Environmental Medicine

This assembly of twenty two concerned medical doctors called for a ban on mobile phone use by small children and restrictions for teens. The reason this "call to action" was so critical was because of the type of diseases they were observing in their patients at unusually accelerated rates. All of which have been shown to be a direct consequence of RF/MW radiation exposure from cell phones and their towers.[251]

- ## The British Medical Association's Board of Science & Education

The British Medical Association's Board of Science & Education has issued a report advising cell phone users to limit their RF/MW radiation exposure, especially when it involves children and their use.[252]

- ## The British Parliament's Independent Expert Group on Mobile Phones / The Stewart Commission

Professor Challis, chairman of the Mobile Telecommunications Health Research Team, has expressed deep concern regarding the extent to which the youth are exploiting the use of cell phones. He believes that more needs to be done to educate our children about limiting the time they spend on their phones.[253]

This assembly, primarily made up of biomedical specialists, joins in supporting the belief that "the widespread use of mobile phones by children for non-essential calls should be discouraged." They also recommended, "That the mobile

---

[251] *The EMR Network.*
http://www.emrpolicy.org/regulation/international/docs/freiburger_appeal.pdf
Also see statements from other countries.
[252] "Mobile Phones and Health," *The British Medical Association's Board of Science & Education,* May 24, 2001.
[253] "The Government Wants Us to Say that These Masts are Completely Safe and Aren't Dangerous, But We Can't Say That," Interview by Andy Mosley, *Express & Echo,* January 24, 2003.

phone industry should refrain from promoting the use of mobile phones by children."[254]

- ## The British Government

  In order to make strides toward addressing the seriousness of children, cell phone use, and their related health hazards, the British Government has recommended that all cell phones carry a warning label advising buyers that the devices should not be used by children.[255]

- ## The French Government

  The French Government has issued a parental advisory to limit children's cell phone use.[256] French officials also gave two additional warnings: They strongly advised pregnant women to distance their cell phones from their bellies and teenagers were instructed to keep cell phones away from their developing sex organs.[257]

  The section on Reproductive Concerns in Chapter 8 addresses several reasons why the French Government may have issued such warnings.

- ## The Australian Senate Environment, Communications, Information Technology and the Arts References Committee [258]

- ## Dr. Lief Salford, Lund University Neurosurgeon, Professor, Author of Multiple RF/MW Studies, and Concerned Father

---

[254] The Independent Expert Group on Mobile Phones, *"Mobile Phones and Health"*, Advice to Industry Vol. 1.No. 53 (April 2000), p. 8.

[255] Carlo, George and Martin Schram, *Cell Phones: Invisible Hazards of the Wireless Age* 2001, Carroll & Graf Publishers New York, NY p. XI

[256] *ACN Online*, "Electrical Sensitivity: A Global Growing Concern. How Wireless Technology May Impact Child Development and Central Nervous System Functioning," Association for Comprehensive Neurotherapy.

[257] "Eye on Europe," *Microwave News*, Vol. 22, No. 2 (March/April 2002) p.5.

[258] Inquiry into Electromagnetic Radiation June 2000. And "Kids Phone Usage Fears," *The Sunday Tasmanian,* March 18, 2001.

- Professor Albert Gjedde,
  Denmark Scientist and Brain Specialist

  Following a study on cell phones and cancer, Gjedde arrived at the conclusion that EMF exposure has the potential to lead to more serious brain damage in children than in adults. He suggested that Denmark reduce their mobile phone exposure to a minimum.[259]

- Olle Johansson,
  Associate Professor, Department of Neuroscience,
  Karolinska Institute in Sweden

  Olle Johansson, respected researcher, has been warning the public about the harmful effects of cell phone microwave irradiation on children since 1996.[260]

- Dr. Om Gandhi,
  One of the First Cell Phone Research Scientists,
  University of Utah, Salt Lake City

  Dr. Gandhi's 1996 study was the first to identify how cell phone radiation affects children to a much greater degree than adults, it could easily be presumed that this highly respected researcher's name be added to this list.

- Dr. Ross Adey,
  One of the World's Most Respected and
  Widely Published Senior Research Experts
  in the area of Health Effects and RF/MW Radiation

  Dr. Adey has spoken out to say that, "Children categorically should not be encouraged or allowed to use" cell phones.[261]

---

[259] Maish, Don, "Mobile Phone Use: It's Time to Take Precautions," *ACNEM Journal,* Vol. 20, No. 1 (April 2001): p. 4.

[260] *ACN Online*, "Electrical Sensitivity: A Global Growing Concern. How Wireless Technology May Impact Child Development and Central Nervous System Functioning," Association for Comprehensive Neurotherapy.

[261] Begich, Nick and Roderick, James, "Cell Phone Convenience or 21st Century Plague?," *Earthpulse Press, Inc.* http://www.earthpulse.com

- Dr. George Carlo,
  Epidemiologist and Wireless Safety Advocate

  "Children under the age of ten should not use wireless devices of any type."[262]

- Dr. Jerry Phillips,
  Research Biochemist

  Dr. Phillips assisted Dr. Adey with the Motorola-funded study which led to the uncovering of DNA damage to human blood cells resulting from mobile phone radiation exposure. After careful evaluation of these and other findings, Phillips made the comment, "I wouldn't let my child play in traffic. I'm not going to give my child a cell phone to put up against her head".[263]

- Dr. Gro Harlem Brundtland,
  General Director of WHO (The World Health Organization), former Prime Minister of Norway, and a Physician with a Degree in Public Health

  Dr. Brundtland discourages children from using mobile phones and likewise advises adults to limit their use and exposure.[264] Brundtland is electro-sensitive and personally suffers from headaches and warmth around the ear whenever she is on her phone. She's discovered what many others have, that contrary to what's believed, making shorter calls doesn't help alleviate the symptoms.[265]

---

[262] George Carlo and Martin Schram, *Cell Phones: Invisible Hazards of the Wireless Age* (New York, NY: Carroll & Graf Publishers, 2001), p. 250.

[263] Kelley, Libby, CWTI (Council on Wireless Technology Impacts), and EON International, DVD *"Public Exposure: DNA, Democracy and the Wireless Revolution"*, 2000.

[264] *ACN Online*, "Electrical Sensitivity: A Global Growing Concern. How Wireless Technology May Impact Child Development and Central Nervous System Functioning," Association for Comprehensive Neurotherapy.

[265] "WHO Director on Cell Phones: Follow Precautionary Principle", *Microwave News*, Vol. 22, No. 2 (March/April 2002): p 6.

- Professor Michael Kundi,
  University of Vienna, Austria

- Physicians for a Healthy Environment in Austria[266]

    In order to educate parents and the general public, Austria's Physicians for a Healthy Environment produced an informational booklet to discourage the use of mobiles among children. Due to the consequences resulting from exposure to cell phone microwave radiation, allowing children to use the device is not only risky; it could lead to an early, preventable death.[267]

- Purachai Piemsomboon,
  The Government Minister of Thailand

    Purachai Piemsomboon has advised teenagers that if they continue to ignore the warning about limiting their cell phone use, a law to ban mobile phone use among teens might become necessary. This cautionary reprimand came after a Japanese study concluded that cell phone radiation causes brain cell and nerve damage, especially in young people.[268]

- The Environment Minister of Bangladesh

    The Environment Minister of Bangladesh has given serious consideration to incorporating a law that would ban the use of mobile phones for those 16 years of age and under. Family members have also been encouraged to keep their phones away from children. National policy is also being considered to restrict companies from selling mobiles to children.[269]

---

[266] *ACN Online*, "Electrical Sensitivity: A Global Growing Concern. How Wireless Technology May Impact Child Development and Central Nervous System Functioning," Association for Comprehensive Neurotherapy.

[267] "More Reasons Children May Be At Risk", *Microwave News,* Vol. 22, No. 4 (July/August 2002): p 13.

[268] "Thai Minister Mulls Cell Phone Ban for Youngsters," Channel News Asia: *Southeast Asia News* April 5, 2002.

[269] "Bangladesh to Ban Mobile Phones for Children," *Ananova-Orange Mobile News Service.* http://www.ananova.com (June 3, 2002).

- Dr. Gerard Hyland,
  Physicist at Warwick University, Coventry, England and the
  International Institute of Biophysics,
  Neuss-Holzheim, Germany

Based on the disturbing evidence revealed in his extensive study of the research, Dr. Hyland had this to say, "If I were a parent I would now be extremely wary about allowing my children to use a mobile even for a very short period. My advice would be to avoid mobiles."[270]

- Gerry Haddad,
  CSIRO Telecommunications
  and Industrial Physics Chief

Standing before the Australian Senate in 2000, Haddad warned that the proposed exposure limits did not take a high enough precautionary level of safety, especially for children. He recommended that the senate "Restrict use of mobile phones to children for essential purposes."[271]

Due to the abundance of information derived from the numerous worldwide efforts of well recognized and respected researchers in this area, it is undeniably obvious that children who use mobiles are posed with a much greater risk than adults. This extensive list of well respected scientists, governments, and other professionals, reflects acceptance of the current data and supports a proactive approach to keep children protected from a very serious health threat.

While these facts, which have repeatedly been confirmed, seem to give enough indication of danger for the French and British governments to take precautionary measures to inform and protect their nation's youth from harm, that's not what's happening here in the United States. The FDA and the FCC have stated that "the scientific evidence does not show a danger to users of wireless

[270] *ACN Online,* "Electrical Sensitivity: A Global Growing Concern. How Wireless Technology May Impact Child Development and Central Nervous System Functioning," Association for Comprehensive Neurotherapy.

[271] The Australian Senate Environment, Communications, Information Technology and the Arts Reference Committee: Inquiry into Electromagnetic Radiation, June 2000. Also: "Kids Phone Usage Fears," *The Sunday Tasmanian,* March 18, 2001.

communication devices, including children." However, they do acknowledge that "some groups sponsored by other national governments have advised that children be discouraged from using wireless phones at all". [272]

Regardless of how these precautionary advisories are viewed by U.S. government officials, these other regimens have made a stand based on their own objective research, not on what they are told by one of the wealthiest and fastest growing industries in the world.

If your children are begging you for a cell phone, talk to them about the risks associated with cell phone use. It will undoubtedly be a challenge to convince them that what you're saying is true, especially when their friends already possess the item in question. However, if even half of what you've learned from this book bubbles to the surface and is recognized as being accurate in the future, as it was with smoking, it will be worth the effort to put off the purchase as long as possible.

Another method of persuasion is to act as if you believe what you're saying. In other words, lead by example; your children want to be just like you (even though in their later years they aren't willing to admit it). When they're young and impressionable, downplay the importance of your phone; when they're older, demonstrate how to use the phone wisely. Helpful tips are provided in the next chapter.

If you're not a parent, but a grandparent, uncle, aunt, teacher, coach, or any other role model that children look up to, don't be afraid to share with them what you've learned from this book. Educate the youngsters who are important to you. They'll listen. It's the "word of mouth" networking that all of us need to get this critical message out to family members, friends, and others we care about. Through our combined effort we can all make a difference in the lives of our children.

---

[272] Quotes found on both the FDA.gov and the FCC.gov websites. Also located in the brochure entitled, "Consumer Information about Radio Frequency Emissions" which accompanies all new cell phones in the U.S..

CHAPTER 12

Playing it Smart

The purpose for writing this book was not to create a panic or to scare you into giving up your cell phone. Nor was it written to make you feel as though you are completely defenseless against this technological form of environmental pollution, also referred to as electrosmog. On the contrary, its intent is to educate and inform you; to tell you what nobody else is telling you, because I strongly believe that you have a right to know all that I've learned through my research and experience. Knowledge is power. With it we can make intelligent decisions; without it we can become extremely vulnerable and can fall victim to that of which we have no understanding.

For cell phone users, ignorance is not bliss. Ignorance has multiple detrimental effects some are even fatal. Once knowledge is acquired, you have to decide what you're going to do with it. You can accept it or reject it. Either way, I strongly advise you to take as many precautionary measures as possible to reduce unnecessary radiation exposure. And do whatever it takes to keep your children safe. Even if you don't believe all that's written in this book, you will have lost nothing by playing it smart.

Ways to Reduce Exposure

➢ Use a Corded, Land Line Phone Whenever Possible.

Phones with cords, although confining and archaic, do not emit harmful radiation or cause any adverse health effect. Therefore, they are a much safer and healthier choice. The FDA and the EPA have both recommended the use of landline phones whenever possible.[273]

While cordless phones are more convenient than corded phones, cordless phones utilize the same RF/MW technology as cell phones to transmit their wireless signals, therefore both can adversely impact your health the same way.

> Limit Your Cell Phone Use.

Cell phones were initially created for emergency purposes only. However, years of industry promotion and the denial of dangers has made cell phones what they are today. Most operators don't give the slightest thought to making a call to talk about nothing.

Now knowing that consequences of long-term use do exist, you are in a better position to gauge the necessity of each call prior to making it or taking it. You are also better equipped to intentionally limit the number and length of your calls.

Dr. Roger Coghill, biologist and British mobile phone specialist has made this comment. "There is overwhelming evidence from 12 laboratories now that excessive use of a mobile phone, such as 20 minutes (a day), could be a serious health risk. Anyone who uses a mobile phone for longer quite literally needs their head examined."[274]

> Keep Calls as Short as Possible
  (preferably under 60 seconds).

Before making a call, identify the purpose for which you are calling. Doing this can help reduce the length of your outgoing calls, keeping them as short as possible, and eliminating unnecessary exposure. Since data indicates that most of the heating effect associated with absorption occurs within the first 60-90 seconds of exposure, it is best to limit calls to 60 seconds or less. Remember that the number of calls you make, *plus* the number of minutes you spend on your phone will determine the likelihood of developing both short and long-term health problems. There's very little

[273] Robert Kane, *Cellular Telephone Russian Roulette* (New York, NY: Vantage Press, 2001), p. 229.
[274] "Mobile Phones Linked to Cancer," *BBC News,* November 9, 1998.

difference between being on the phone for several short calls and being on the phone for a few long calls.

> ## Distance Your Cell Phone from Your Body.

The distance between your cell phone and your body determines the level of radiation exposure and absorption you will experience. Exposure is reduced the farther away your phone is from your body. Likewise, exposure increases the closer it is to your body. Simply put, there's really only one key word you need to remember in order to play it smart: *Distance*.

While everyone seems to have their cell phone attached to their belt or in their front pant's pocket while their phone is in "standby" mode, this is an unwise decision. Cell phones carried or worn near the waist in this manner operate at higher power levels than normal because the tissue and the organs in that particular region (the liver, the kidney, and the testes) absorb more radiation than other body parts. This increased absorption makes the phone work harder, receiving and emitting greater amounts of radiation, in order to maintain a strong signal.[275] Increased absorption intensifies heating, which destroys cells and causes damage.

Since the heart is so vulnerable and breast tissue is recognized as having an accelerated absorption rate when exposed to RF/MW energy, transporting cell phones against the chest is also highly unadvisable. The extent, to which business men are carrying their cell phones in their suit pocket, resting it against their chest, could be contributing to the growing incidents of breast cancer in men. Based on all of the information that has been disclosed in this publication, cell phone operators who tote their phones on their bodies in "standby" mode are asking for trouble. They are posed with consequences too great to minimize. Just on the lower portion of their body they can expect to experience an increased risk of liver and testicular cancer. Men exposed to this type of close range cell phone radiation are also likely to experience a reduction of testosterone, problematic erections, up to a 30% decrease in sperm count, and a significant reduction of sperm quality.[276, 277, 278, 279]

---

[275] "Cell Phone On Your Belt Brings Radiation to the Liver and Kidneys," *The Sunday Mirror*, July 10, 1999.

[276] Fejes, Imre, et al., *"Relationship Between Regular Cell Phone Use and Human Semen Quality,"* paper presented at the 20th Annual Meeting of the European Society of Human Reproduction and Embryology, Berlin, June 29, 2004.

Women electing to wear cell phones against their bodies are more likely to develop cervical and breast cancers, both of which have been attributed to RF/MW radiation exposure. [280] And although there's no supporting documentation of this adverse repercussion, I have been told by a number of women that soon after they began carrying their cell phone on their belt, they started having irregular menstrual cycles. Even though millions of people are wearing their cell phones against their body, can you think of one benefit that outweighs maintaining your good health?

> Avoid Holding the Phone Against Your Head.

Instead of having concentrated doses of microwaves radiating deep into your brain, where they are absorbed and cause damage, it's imperative to distance yourself from your phone and its harmful emissions. In Motorola's information pamphlet which accompanies each of their new phones, this advice is given. "Do not hold the unit such that the antenna is exposed to parts of the body when the unit is turned on." Who are they kidding? Unlike the retractable antennas on older models, which allowed you to pull the radiating device away from your head, manufacturers now incorporate the antenna, the most dangerous part of your phone, inside of the phone so it's even closer to your head. What's worse is that all service providers advertise and display pictures of people holding a cell phone tightly pressed against their head, while at the same time the phone's manufacturer is clearly advising you to do just the opposite!

Realizing that the manufacturer is advising operators not to expose an active phone (with an internal antenna) to the body while it's on provides yet another compelling argument against choosing to wear a cell phone against the body when it is in "standby" mode.

---

[277] Lai, Henry, *"Biological Effects of Radiofrequency Radiation"*, Paper for the Scientific Workshop "EMF-Scientific and Legal Issues, Theory and Evidence of EMF Biological and Health Effects" in Catania, Sicily, Italy, September 13-14, 2002, organized by the Italian National Institute for Prevention and Work Safety.

[278] Wayne Rash, "Cell Phone Use Affects Fertility, Study Shows," *EWeek.com*, October 27, 2006.

[279] "Cell Phones Can Affect Sperm Quality, Researcher Says," *CNN News,* September 18, 2008.

[280] Cherry, Neil, *"Cell Phone Radiation Poses a Serious Biological and Health Risk,"* http://www.buergerwelle.de/pdf/cell_phone_radiation_poses_a_serious_biological_and_health_risk.pdf (May 7, 2001).

> ## Keep the Phone Away from Your Head While Connections are Being Made.

Holding the phone away from your head while a call is being made and the signals are connecting is another way of playing it smart. Prior to calls being joined together, the phone's power level is significantly increased in order to achieve complete transmission. To avoid this elevated degree of unnecessary exposure, instead of pressing the phone to your head listening to it ring and waiting for an answer, listen through the speakerphone or watch until your phone's screen indicates that the connection is complete. Any amount of distance created between your head and the phone is better than none.

> ## Use the Speakerphone Whenever Possible.

Opting to use the speakerphone feature whenever possible is another easy way to reduce emissions. The speakerphone enables you to comfortably converse while distancing the cell phone from your head.

> ## Opt for Text Messaging or E-Mailing.

Another means of reducing exposure by creating distance between your head and your phone is to text message or e-mail, rather than talk. If you've got a brief message to communicate, use one of these two methods. Texting and e-mailing both reduce exposure while eliminating unnecessary talk time. If your children own a cell phone, encourage them to use one of these methods to communicate more safely with friends and family.

> ## Alternate Head Sides When Talking on Wireless Phones.

If for some reason you choose to continue holding a cell phone directly against your head, alternate ears while conversing. Data extracted from several studies has shown that those who have used a cell phone for 10+ years are posed with a higher risk of developing brain tumors and acoustic neuromas. The risk of developing a brain tumor for those who alternate head sides while talking on a cell phone is 20%. Those who don't rotate sides, increase their brain tumor risk by 200%! Cell phone users of 3+

years have a 30-60% chance of developing acoustic neuroma.[281] That risk increases to 240% if the cell phone is primarily used on only one side of the head. [282] The same proves true for cordless phones. Get in the habit of switching sides, it's a simple safeguard.

> ➤ Avoid Using Wired Headsets.

Headsets which use metal wiring leading into the ear piece can increase exposure. Instead of reducing the amount of RF/MW radiation being absorbed into your head, this type of headset actually brings it much closer to your brain than if you had your handset pressed against your ear. The wire not only acts as part of the antenna, the most dangerous part of the phone, but according to the British Consumers Association these popular headsets have been found to deliver 3.5 times as much radiation as handsets. Wired headsets also have the capability of picking up other concentrated electromagnetic fields (EMFs) from nearby sources, thereby contributing even more intensified amounts of radiation into the user's head.[283]

> ➤ Avoid Using Wireless Ear Pieces.

Similarly, wireless ear pieces should be avoided. These innovative hands-free devices operate at the same frequency level as cell phones, utilizing identical RF/MW technology. However, they are much more dangerous because instead of limiting your exposure to when you're actually using your phone, these contraptions hang on your ear in "standby" mode, constantly receiving and transmitting signals to and from nearby cell sites. This same chronic exposure is why it's best to avoid wearing your cell phone on or against your body.

---

[281] George Carlo and Martin Schram, *Cell Phones: Invisible Hazards of the Wireless Age* (New York, NY: Carroll & Graf Publishers, 2001), p. 170.
[282] Sage, C., *The Bio Initiative Report,*
http://www.bioinitiative.org/report/docs/section_1.pdf (May 2008), p. 9.
[283] "The Invisible Dangers of EMF Radiation", *BioPro International, Inc.,* http://www.biopro.com (March 22, 2005).

> Refrain from Using Your Cell Phone while Driving.

While most drivers believe that they can successfully drive and talk on their cell phone at the same time, research efforts prove otherwise. Frequently, cell phone users drive with just one hand on the steering wheel, they are easily distracted by their conversations, and their focus is not on the road. Evidence of neurological effects that hinder driving include a reduced awareness of surroundings, a decreased capacity for paying attention, slower reaction times along with an inability to make quick decisions and respond to them accordingly. As exemplified by a University of Utah study, these impairments are equivalent to those of a drunk driver. [284]

Other neurological abnormalities linked to exposure that could affect driving include increased levels of stress, anxiety, and irritability. On the road this could easily translate into the agitated behavior some refer to as "road rage".

Two studies, one conducted by the University of Toronto in Canada and the other by The Insurance Institute for Highway Safety in Perth, Australia, both resolved that cell phone users are 4 times as likely to get into a serious car accident than other drivers.[285] It has also been reported that cell phone operators who use their phone for 50+ minutes a day, while driving or not, are 5.6 times as likely to get into an automobile accident than those who are on their phone less often.[286] Not only do the number of accidents increase with heightened levels of exposure, but the degree of severity and fatality probability is also significantly elevated.[287]

Due to this noticeable hazard, many states have made it illegal to drive while holding a handset. To improve your driving ability as well as minimizing your accident risk, you can incorporate the use of a hands free speaker phone, place an external antenna on the outside of your vehicle, or employ the use of an air (not a wired or wireless) headset. All offer safer alternatives to holding a handset to your head while driving.

---

[284] Mitchell, C. L., et al., "Some Behavioral Effects of Short-Term Exposure of Rats to 2.45 GHz Microwave radiation," *Bioelectromagnetics,* Vol. 9, No. 3 (1988): pp. 259-268

[285] Slesin, Louis, *Microwave News* March/April 1997. p. 8.

[286] Violanti, J.M. and Marshall, J.R., "Cellular Phones and Traffic Accidents: An Epidemiological Approach," *Accid Anal Prev* Vol. 28, No.2 (1996): pp. 265-270.

[287] Violanti, J.M., "Cellular Phones and Fatal Traffic Accidents," *Accid Anal Prev Vol.* 30, No. 4 (1998): pp. 519-524.

> ➤ Avoid Using Cell Phones Near Reflective Surfaces.

This may sound rather peculiar to you, but if at all possible avoid using cell phones near reflective surfaces. Studies have shown that your phone's electromagnetic waves, in close proximity to reflective surfaces, can significantly magnify RF/MW radiation exposure. The increased exposure resulting from this reflective effect is at an absorption rate of 4.7 times greater than if proximity to such reflective materials is avoided.[288] This is in addition to the 50-90% which is already being absorbed into the brain from your phone's energy. This concept is similar to that of using a sun reflector to intensify exposure while sunbathing.[289]

Also, if you use your phone while driving, be aware that inside your vehicle you are surrounded by numerous reflective, metal components. These intensify your level of exposure, maximizing the heating effect, as well as your rate of radiation absorption. Other places of excessive exposure include office buildings, elevators, subways, trains, airplanes, and the like, which are constructed primarily of metal. Unfortunately, your cell phone is not the only culprit; other people's cell phones, wireless networks, and nearby cell towers also play an active and considerable role in the amount of irradiation you receive from reflective surroundings.

Studies have also found evidence that cell phone users who wear metal-framed glasses significantly increase their eye exposure by 20% and their head exposure by 6.3%.[290] Since this seemingly insignificant reflective article magnifies and accelerates exposure, it would stand to reason that people with braces or those who wear reflective jewelry can also be imperiled to a heightened degree.

---

[288] O. P Gandhi, et al, "Deposition of Electromagnetic Energy in Animals and in Models of Man with and without Grounding and Reflector Effects, *Radio Science,* November/December 1977, pp. 39-47.

[289] Robert Kane, *Cellular Telephone Russian Roulette* (New York, NY: Vantage Press, 2001), pp. 59, 158.

[290] House of Commons, Great Britain. Third Report, The Science and Technology Committee. *"Scientific Advisory System: Mobile Phones and Health,"* September 22, 1999.

➤ Keep Cell Phones "OFF" When Not in Use.

Keeping your phone "off" (absent of signal) when it's not in use minimizes exposure. Rather than leaving it "on" in "standby" mode when you're not making or expecting a call, take advantage of voicemail. Forwarding calls to an available land line is also a beneficial option.

➤ Distance Yourself from Other Cell Phone Users.

As you know, distance is necessary in order to avoid unnecessary exposure. Not only is it advisable to maintain distance from your own cell phone, but it's recommended that you maintain your distance from other cell phones as well. Keep this in mind when someone next to you or behind you is using a cell phone in close proximity. The farther you are from the user, the safer you'll be.

➤ Avoid Using Cell Phones in Close Proximity to Small Children.

This is important enough to repeat. Children have an elevated risk of radiation absorption and potential damage from exposure, so it's critical to be aware of their propinquity while talking on your phone. If you notice that you're too close, simply step away. Remember, the smaller the child, the greater the risk.

➤ Avoid Using Cell Phones when Signal Strength is Weak.

Cell phone operation is least hazardous when signal strength is strong. When the phone has a powerful signal it doesn't have to work as hard and emits less energy. Therefore, prior to making or taking a call, determine your phone's signal strength. The closer you are to the nearest tower or base station the stronger your signal will be, and the farther away you are, the weaker the signal.

When you have a weak signal, your phone has to work harder and use more power to make a call. The harder your phone has to work to transmit or receive a signal, the more radiation is required. To avoid unnecessary exposure only use your phone when signal strength is strong.[291]

---

[291] Slesin, Louis, *Microwave News,* http://microwavenews.com/nc_apr2007.html (April 2007).

➢ Discourage Children & Teens from Using Cell Phones.

Share with your children what you have learned regarding cell phone dangers and encourage them to text message or e-mail friends, rather than calling them. When calls are made, promote speaker phone use. If a land line is available, encourage its use by designating the land line as the first and best option for talking with someone.

➢ Pregnant Women Should Avoid Cell Phone Use Entirely.

Pregnant women should avoid being unnecessarily exposed to all types of wireless signals, not just cell phone signals. Wearing a cell phone on the body while pregnant should be avoided at all costs, because exposure to this kind of radiation has been shown to result in miscarriage, birth defects, and all sorts of damage to the unborn child.

➢ Give your Brain a Break.

Give your brain a break after each phone call. Recovery time can vary from one mobile conversation to another. The length of the call should be indicative as to the amount of repair time necessary. Longer exposures constitute longer repair time and shorter exposures need less time. Without the ability to feel or see actual cell and tissue damage, it's difficult to know how much time is enough.

Bear in mind that the effects of RF/MW radiation are cumulative; repeated damage from several shorts calls or a few long calls without adequate recovery time can result in permanent, long-term consequences.

➢ Take Other Precautionary Measures.

If you choose to use a cell phone as your primary means of telecommunication or for extensive use, protect yourself from unnecessary exposure and potential harm as much as possible. These safety tips are meant to assist you in keeping safe and playing it smart. Employ as many of them as possible and educate others to do the same.

CONCLUSION

What Now?

If history has taught us anything it is that when new consumer products, offering enormous benefits and having mass appeal emerge into the marketplace, they are eagerly embraced and employed with great enthusiasm and little concern. This is especially true of wireless technology.

While most consumer products introduced for use are FDA-approved and pose no threat of harm, others have later been found to be extremely toxic and carcinogenic. Consider the examples of DDT, lead-based paint, asbestos, and cigarettes. When these items first became available to consumers, sales and use soared without restraint. After decades of exposure to these particular substances people began to get sick and die. These incidents commenced long before the government and the industries manufacturing and selling these products were willing to accept the scientific evidence proving danger as being conclusive and irrefutable. Only then were changes made.

Industry concealment is not an unusual business tactic when the truth threatens to impact the bottom line. "The U.S. government and the asbestos industry have been criticized for not acting quickly enough to inform the public of dangers, and to reduce public exposure. In the late 1970s, court documents proved that asbestos industry officials knew of asbestos dangers and tried to conceal them."[292] An effective concealment of truth was also systematically uncovered when the tobacco industry was finally exposed.

Today we are facing yet another trade organization that is exposing consumers to life-threatening health hazards, yet like the

---

[292] *Wikipedia, The Free Encyclopedia,* http://www.en.wikipedia.org/wiki/Asbestos

others, they are unwilling to inform the public of suspected and recognized dangers. Even though intelligence documents prove that western governments have known that cell phone radiation causes brain damage for more than 30 years, they have hidden the facts proving it![293] Chapter 2 fully exposes other successful industry cover ups.

What we have learned from these lessons is that big business is politically supported and that the denial of facts and research data can be conveniently hidden in order to insure self-preservation. It isn't until the problems become so great and the issue can no longer be contained, that the truth is finally made public. Until then, we remain vulnerable and industries such as these continue to defend their position of safety using the key phrases that were effectively employed by the tobacco industry for decades. "There is not enough evidence proving harm. The studies are inconclusive. More research needs to be done." The question is how long are you willing to wait? How much are you willing to risk?

I hope you found this book to be informative. If you haven't noticed by now, like the cell phone industry, I've developed a belief system of my own. And even while the cellular industry would deem that the evidence remains inconclusive, there are more studies proving adverse health effects than studies proving safety. There is far too much data and supporting documentation from reliable, credible sources to deny that this energy does have a consequential impact on the human body.

While you may be thinking to yourself, "I've been using a cell phone for years and nothing bad is happening to me." Just know that the effects of RF/MW radiation exposure are rarely immediate, they are cumulative. It's not uncommon for toxic reactions to subtly creep in and lay dormant long before a problem is realized. As with all carcinogens, there are comparable manifestations of the irritant, yet every person's body is different with varying tolerance levels. Factors which determine individual reactions include age, health condition, genetic make-up, skull thickness, head shape and size, internal brain structure, hydration and density of tissue. Source of exposure, frequency, waveform, duration of exposure, number of

---

[293] Moran, Kathy, "Soviet Proof That Mobile Phones Do Cause Brain Damage," *Daily Express*, November 10,1999.

exposures, and pulse modulation of the signal also contribute to establishing individual response. [294]

And although it may be no big deal that you forgot to pick your daughter up from piano practice, missed an important meeting, or can't remember the name of an old college friend, a neurological disorder could be developing. Memory loss is not normal neither are headaches, concentration difficulties, sleeping problems, dizziness, mood swings, irritability, anxiety or fatigue. If these abnormalities persist and are ignored or masked with drugs, they can become irreversible and permanent disorders which can lead to life-threatening diseases.

As you go forth in your search for answers, every time new information becomes available give the most consideration to studies that are conducted by independent, non-interested, third-party researchers and organizations. These offer an elevated degree of credibility, because objective views can't be bought.

One thing is for certain, change is needed in order to ensure safety. We can no longer remain quiet. We must speak out. In the United States, hundreds of cell towers, along with multitudes of other wireless networks, such as Wi-Fi and WI-MAX, are being erected daily. As the desire for newer technology increases, the industry eagerly accommodates by accelerating its expansion. These networks create an environmental hazard and we are all inadvertently and involuntarily being exposed to higher and more dangerous levels of RF/MW radiation. There appears to be no end to this escalation in sight, but the adoption of a more reasonable safety standard is a realistic measure that can be taken in order to help protect society and preserve quality of life.

Even if only half of what's written in this book is true, shouldn't it motivate you to take a proactive approach to your cell phone use? Continuing to use your wireless wonder freely and without restraint, assuming it's safe and throwing all caution to the wind, is downright foolish. Don't wait until it's too late. Ignoring the facts doesn't change them.

---

[294] Sage, C., *The Bio Initiative Report,*
http://www.bioinitiative.org/report/docs/section_1.pdf (May 2008), p. 14.

Glossary of Terms

Athermal
Non-thermal. Any effect from electromagnetic energy which is not heat induced.

Base Station
An antenna structure which relays wireless RF/MW radiation signals between phones and other wireless devices to make and maintain connections.

Blood Brain Barrier (BBB)
A protective membrane and filtering system lining the exterior of the brain. Its function is to restrict the entrance of harmful toxins from entering the bloodstream and reaching the brain.

Carcinogen
Any substance that produces cancer.

CRADA (Cray-da)
Cooperative Research and Development Agreement. An agreement between the federal government and the industry to collectively do research.

CTIA
Cellular Telecommunications Internet Association. Formerly known as the Cellular Telecommunications Industry Association. The trade organization that represents wireless service providers.

Electrosensitivity, Electromagnetic Hypersensitivity
Unusual and often painful responses leading to adverse health effects from exposure to electric, magnetic or electromagnetic fields (EMFs).

Electromagnetic Field (EMF)
The generic term for the radiation that emanates from devices that operate using electric currents or radio waves.

Electromagnetic Radiation (EMR)
Oscillating electric and magnetic fields which can be classified as either ionizing or non-ionizing, based on whether it is capable of electrically charging atoms and breaking chemical bonds.

Electromagnetic Spectrum
Encompasses the range of all electromagnetic radiation from below the frequencies used for radio (long waves), to microwaves, infrared, visible, ultraviolet, x-ray, through to gamma radiation (short waves).

ELF
Extra low or extremely low frequency.

EPA
U.S. Environmental Protection Agency.

Epidemiology
Studies of diseases conducted on human groups and populations.

FCC
U.S. Federal Communications Commission. The branch of government which oversees all communication development and technology. It also sets acceptable criteria and parameters.

FDA
Food and Drug Administration. This U.S. branch of government is responsible for protecting citizens from all products that will be used by consumers.

Frequency
The number of oscillations or cycles per unit of time; cycles completed by electromagnetic waves in 1 second are usually expressed in hertz (Hz). Wireless communication signals operate at different frequencies.

GSM
Global System for Mobile communication. A digital, wireless network.

Hertz (Hz)
The speed in which radio waves travel. One hertz equates to one cycle per second.

Ionizing Radiation
Short electromagnetic waves which contain sufficient speed and energy to electrically charge ions and break chemical bonds (disconnecting electrons from atoms).

Megahertz (MHz)
A million cycles per second, radio wave speed.

Micronuclei
An abnormality of DNA fragments indicating genetic damage.

Microwaves
Non-ionizing mini short waves which are part of the electromagnetic spectrum. Microwaves are used to transmit and receive wireless signals.

Non-Ionizing Radiation
Short electromagnetic waves that do not contain sufficient speed or energy to electrically charge ions and break chemical bonds. Typically, non-ionizing radiation does not produce external heating, but it can elicit an undetectable heating response deep within biological tissue.

Power Density
The amount of power which is emitted from an electromagnetic wave at any given point. Measured in watts per square meter. A signal's power density weakens as distance from the source increases.

Radiofrequency (RF)
Rate of oscillation in electrical circuits or electromagnetic radiation within the range of 3 Hz to 300 GHz.

Radiofrequency Microwave (RF/MW) Radiation
The non-ionizing energy used to transmit and receive wireless signals.

Specific Absorption Rate (SAR)
How standards are established. The calculation used to determine how much RF energy is absorbed into 1 cubic gram of human tissue over a specified period of time. It is measured in watts per kilogram (W/kg). In the U.S., the allowable SAR from cell phones is 1.6 W/kg. Whole body exposure is not to exceed 0.8 W/kg averaged over 30 minutes.

WHO
World Health Organization.

Wi-Fi
Wireless Fidelity. A trademark of the Wi-Fi Alliance which certifies residential and commercial networks, mobile phones, video games, and other devices that require wireless networking. The term Wi-Fi is commonly used to depict *all* wireless Internet (WLAN) connections, regardless of whether or not they are actually Wi-Fi certified. Signals can transmit as far as 6 miles.

WiMAX Wireless Networks
Similar to WiFi networks, but these signals operate at higher speeds and can cover radial distances of up to 30 miles.[295]

Wireless Technology Research, L.L.C. (WTR)
A legal entity established by the CTIA to oversee industry-funded research efforts examining health impacts on the human body from wireless RF/MW radiation.

W/kg
Watts per kilogram. A unit of measurement used to determine SAR.

WLAN
Wireless Local Area Network used to establish Internet connections.

Definitions were extracted from a combination of Wikopedia.com, Carlo, George and Martin Schram, *Cell Phones: Invisible Hazards of the Wireless Age* (New York, NY: Carroll & Graf Publishers, 2001), pp. 262-265, and the glossary of terms from Sage, C., *The Bio Initiative Report,*
http://www.bioinitiative.org/report/docs/section_1.pdf (May 2008).
[295] Brain, Marshall, and Ed Grabianowski. "How WiMAX Works." 02 December 2004. HowStuffWorks.com. http://computer.howstuffworks.com/wimax.htm 16 February 2009.

Thank you for investing in this book. I hope you found it to be eye-opening and thought-provoking. Knowledge empowers us with the ability to make wise decisions. Proverbs 2:11 promises that discretion will protect you and understanding will guard you.

Is someone you love always on their cell phone? Isn't it time they realized the consequences of their excessive exposure, before it's too late? This book makes a great gift idea, one that shows how much you care. Buy it online today at **www.RealCellPhoneDangers.com** both paperback and e-book versions are available. You are also invited to submit your feedback and comments, shop our store of RF-reducing products, and get updated information on research about cell phone dangers and other wireless issues as they emerge.

If you consider this information valuable, please share what you've learned with your family and friends. Email them a link to **www.RealCellPhoneDangers.com** so that they can also become empowered with knowledge to make wise decisions regarding their exposure and that of their family. They will genuinely appreciate it.

Wholesale pricing, affiliate opportunities, and drop-shipping are available. Submit all inquiries to Premier Advantage Publishing.

➢ the web site:
  www.PremierAdvantagePublishing.com
  or www.RealCellPhoneDangers.com

➢ email:
  contactus@premieradvantagepublishing.com

➢ direct mail:
  Premier Advantage Publishing
  3819 Rivertown Pkwy, Ste. 300-#210
  Grandville, MI 49418   USA

➢ phone:
  248.747-8234

Carleigh Cooper's mission is to educate cell phone users on the real dangers which are proven to exist as a direct result of wireless RF/MW radiation exposure. Carleigh is available for book signings, speaking engagements, personal interviews, and other public relations events. For more information, please contact Premier Advantage Publishing, using one of the above methods.